SECRETS OF
SHIATSU

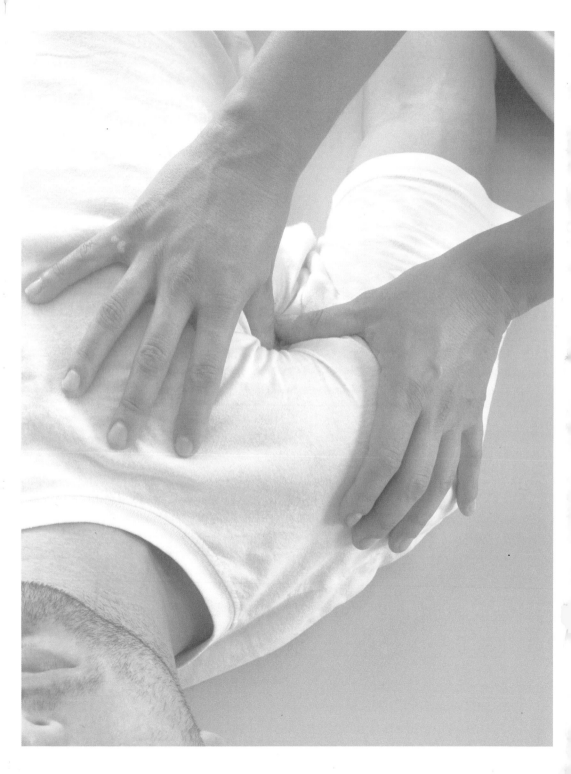

SECRETS OF
SHIATSU

CATHY MEEUS

CONSULTANT
PAUL LUNDBERG

IVY PRESS

This edition published in the UK and North America in 2018 by
Ivy Press
An imprint of The Quarto Group
The Old Brewery, 6 Blundell Street
London N7 9BH, United Kingdom
T (0)20 7700 6700 **F** (0)20 7700 8066
www.QuartoKnows.com

First published in 2000

© 2017 Quarto Publishing plc

British Library Cataloguing-in-Publication Data
A catalogue record for this book is available from the British Library

ISBN: 978-1-78240-574-0

This book was conceived, designed and produced by
Ivy Press
58 West Street, Brighton BN1 2RA, United Kingdom
Art director Peter Bridgewater
Editorial Director Sophie Collins
Design Manager Anna Stevens
Designers Kevin Knight, Jane Lanaway, Ginny Zeal
Editor Rowan Davies, Sara Harper
Picture Researcher Liz Eddison, Vanessa Fletcher, Alison Stevens
Photography Guy Ryecart
Photography administration Kay MacMullan
Illustrations Sarah Young, Anna Hunter-Downing, Coral Mula,
Rhian Nest-James, Andrew Milne, Catherine McIntyre, Ivan Hissey
Three-dimensional models Mark Jamieson

Printed in China

10 9 8 7 6 5 4 3 2 1

Note from the publisher
Although every effort has been made to ensure that the information
presented in this book is correct, the authors and publisher cannot
be held responsible for any injuries which may arise.

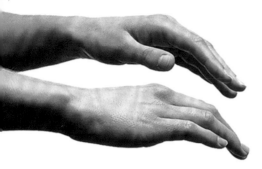

Finger work

The Japanese word
"shiatsu" is translated as
"finger pressure."

HOW TO USE THIS BOOK To make this book simple to

use, it is divided into sections giving either information or practical instructions. Concise background information about the shiatsu techniques is followed by easy-to-follow step-by-step guides illustrated with color photographs. The book takes you through the principles behind this ancient therapy, then introduces preparation for shiatsu and basic techniques. The core of the book concentrates on a basic shiatsu routine and then the final section outlines shiatsu self-help treatments for common ailments.

Important Notice

Do not use shiatsu to replace medical treatment you are receiving for any significant health problem. If you are in any doubt about the suitability of shiatsu for your condition, please seek the advice of your doctor before practicing these exercises, or receiving treatment. Always observe the cautions, particularly if you are pregnant, or have high blood pressure, or epilepsy.

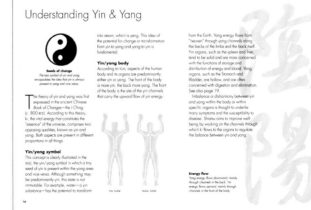

Background knowledge

The principles and philosophy behind shiatsu are
explained at the beginning of the book.

SHOULDER & ARM ROTATION The first stage mobilizes the shoulder joint to open the channels that pass through it and facilitates the free flow of energy between the arm and body. Stretching the arm both vertically and forward further relaxes and opens the shoulder area. Increase the stretches only gradually, working from your hara and looking out for indications of discomfort from the receiver. Your supporting hand is especially important because the shoulder is a complex joint.

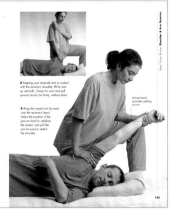

3 Keeping your nearside arm in contact with the receiver's shoulder, lift his arm up vertically. Grasp his wrist and pull upward slowly but firmly, without strain.

4 Bring the raised arm forward over the receiver's head. Adjust the position of the passive hand to stabilize the armpit, and pull the arm forward to stretch the shoulder.

Active hand provides pulling action

1 Support the front of the shoulder with the hand that is nearest the receiver. Place your other hand on his back, over the shoulder blade.

2 Hold the shoulder with both hands and rotate the shoulder a few times in each direction. Use the movement from your hara, not just your arms, to direct the rotation.

142   143

Practical

Practical color spreads detail the stances and step-by-step guides to specific shiatsu routines.

Side Position

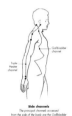

Side channels
The principal channels accessed from the side of the body are the Gallbladder and Triple Heater.

The main part of the basic routine ends with the receiver lying on his or her side. This position allows you to gain access to the Triple Heater and Gallbladder channels. Sections of the Liver and Heart Protector channels, which

have not previously been worked, are also reached easily.

Triple Heater
The Triple Heater channel distributes energy in three areas of the body known as the Upper, Middle, and Lower Heater regions, harmonizing the activities of the organs in those areas. Much of the activity of this "organ" is concerned with the processing and transportation of fluids. In the Upper Heater, fluids are transformed into vapor. Nourishing fluids are transported throughout the body from the Middle Heater. The Lower Heater processes and eliminates waste fluids. This concern with fluids provides a close link with the activities of the Kidneys. The Triple Heater also plays an important defensive role against environmental factors, such as cold and infection, leading to an association with the immune system. Shiatsu treatment of the Triple Heater channel gives an overall boost to the system, promoting the healthy flow of energy from the Kidneys throughout the body, providing a sense of warmth and well-being.

Gallbladder
The Gallbladder channel plays a key role in digestion and purposeful mental activity and works in close association with the Liver. Disturbance of these channels may lead to indigestion, joint and muscle stiffness, and frustration and indecision. Working on these channels enhances mental agility and creativity, as well as physiological functions.

Heart Protector
Working the Heart Protector channel benefits heart and circulatory function. It can also have tremendous mental and emotional effects, helping to overcome shyness or caution.

Before starting work, check that the receiver is comfortable, with the top leg bent and resting in front to provide stability. Use a pillow under the head and another under the knee and thigh of the bent leg. Choose a kneeling or half-kneeling position that enables you to complete the stretches without strain. Complete the entire routine (see pages 142–59) on one side of the body before asking the receiver to turn over.

140   141

Detail

Each color spread is supplemented by more detailed information on each aspect of shiatsu.

TREATMENT ROUTINE When back pain is acute (of recent onset), rest is way to allow the muscles time to relax, and to permit depleted ki to be replenished — an important aspect of recovery. While you rest, have a helper work on tsubos away from your back. When pain has abated, have shiatsu treatment of the back itself. In the long term, examine your lifestyle to prevent a recurrence of the problem.

Back strengthening
Regular work on the tsubos of the Bladder channel located on the foot—B.62 and B.60— is often effective for strengthening the back after strain or injury. B.40, at the back of the knee, is a well-known tsubo for helping the back to withstand strain.

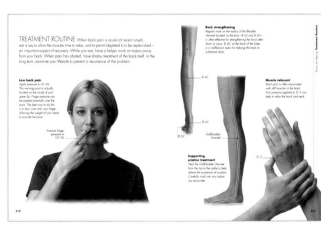

Low back pain
Apply pressure to GV 26. This reviving point is actually located on the inside of your upper lip. Finger pressure can be exerted externally over the point. The best way to do this is to lean over onto your finger, allowing the weight of your head to provide the force.

External finger pressure to GV 26

B.40

B.60

B.62

Gallbladder channel

Supporting sciatica treatment
Treat the Gallbladder channel from the hip to the ankle to help relieve the symptoms of sciatica. Carefully untie any tsubos you encounter.

Muscle relaxant
Back pain is often associated with stiff muscles in the back. Firm pressure applied at SI 3 can help to relax the back and neck.

SI 3

210   211

Self-help

The final section of the book details self-help routines you can carry out to help alleviate the symptoms of common ailments.

Introduction: From the Yellow Emperor to Masunaga

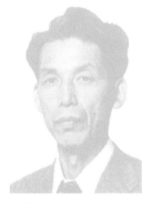

Shizuto Masunaga
The author of Zen Shiatsu, *and the leading exponent of the branch of shiatsu that inspires this book.*

Shiatsu, meaning "finger pressure," is a modern bodywork therapy that arose out of an Eastern healing tradition dating back thousands of years. The first expression of Chinese medical theories appears in *The Yellow Emperor's Classic of Internal Medicine* (c. 100 BCE). This ancient work lays out the basis of diagnosis and treatment, including the therapeutic use of points stimulation by needle, massage, and heat.

Theories

The Chinese healing tradition was well established in Japan by the sixth century ad, where *anma*, the Japanese form of *anmo* (acupuncture and massage), was widely practiced. However, this practice declined until the early twentieth century, when the pioneering work of Tamai Tempaku brought traditional Japanese bodywork back into the mainstream. His book *Shiatsu Ho* (1919) inspired later practitioners, such as Tokujiro Namikoshi, Katsusuke Serizawa, and Shizuto Masunaga, influential shiatsu teachers who each developed different practical and theoretical aspects.

Zen shiatsu

Masunaga published *Zen Shiatsu* in 1977. In this he described the system of shiatsu upon which this book primarily draws. Zen shiatsu employs a variety of techniques for manipulating energy flow in the body. The underlying theory is based on Traditional Chinese Medicine, and draws together different strands of the tradition, including *yin* and *yang* and meridian (channel) theory.

The Five Elements

The ancient Five Element theory (see pages 16–19 and pages 20–23) makes further contributions to create a comprehensive system for improving health and combating disease.

Shiatsu has proved increasingly popular in the West, where its holistic approach to treating the person, not the disease, has caught people's imaginations.

Shiatsu & Acupressure

The practice of shiatsu includes the use of many different techniques to influence the body's energy systems. Acupressure, the application of finger pressure to specific points on the body, is one of these. It uses the points (called *tsubos*) identified by acupuncture theory and may be described as "no-needle acupuncture." Some shiatsu practitioners emphasize acupressure work; others rely to a greater extent on other forms of pressure, stretches, or manipulation.

THE PRINCIPLES OF
SHIATSU

Modern shiatsu is a holistic therapy, firmly rooted in Traditional Chinese Medicine and based on the idea that vital energy, known as ki (or qi), flows through channels (sometimes called meridians) in the body. These can be influenced by applying pressure to specific points along the channels, clearing blockages in energy flow, and thereby promoting healthier functioning of specific body systems and of the body as a whole. The therapy is mainly used to regulate the healthy body and to prevent illness. But shiatsu therapy can also be used to address specific health problems, by emphasizing treatment of certain points or areas.

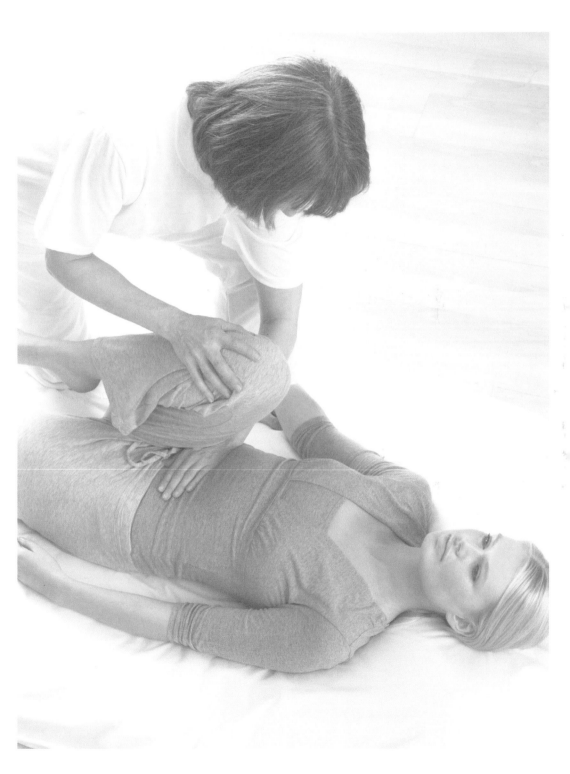

Ideas of Energy

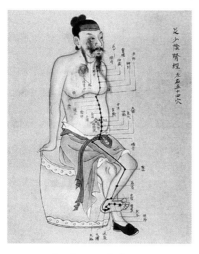

Ancient wisdom
References to energy pathways, meridians, or channels that are used in shiatsu have been found in ancient Chinese manuscripts.

n ancient Chinese philosophy all physical matter in the universe is made up of energy called *qi* (pronounced "chee"). In Japan and in shiatsu theory, qi is known as ki. Ki, sometimes described as the "life force" or "vital energy," can be either material, that is, with a physical form, or nonmaterial. Blood, for example, is seen in TCM as a material form of ki, which nourishes the body's tissues. Ki is manifested in a variety of qualities and aspects, which are defined and elaborated in yin and yang theory (see pages 16–19) and the Five Elements system (see pages 20–23). In the Indian Ayurvedic tradition, there is a similar concept of energy termed *prana*, or breath. Modern Western medicine has no parallel notion of vital energy, but this aspect of the philosophy underlying shiatsu comes close to the theories of subatomic physics.

Life force

According to the theory of Traditional Chinese Medicine (TCM), there are three categories of ki within the body: prenatal or original ki—which is derived from your genetic inheritance; grain ki—which is obtained from food; and air ki—which is gathered from the air you breathe.

The unimpeded flow of ki through the body, like that of the blood supply, is essential to health. It nourishes, restores, and invigorates every part. Conversely, when ki is lacking or the flow is blocked, the functioning of the affected organ is impaired, leading to stagnation and the buildup of toxins. Symptoms of ill health are the likely result.

Vital organs

In TCM the role of the vital organs is viewed very differently than in the Western tradition. The main organs in TCM are the Lungs, Large Intestine, Stomach, Spleen, Heart, Small Intestine, Bladder, Kidneys, Heart Protector (Pericardium), Gallbladder, and Liver. These are ascribed a much wider role than the limited physiological functions recognized by Western medicine. An additional organ exists that has no physical form or anatomical parallel: the Triple Heater (or Triple Burner). Each organ governs a range of physical and emotional states. The specific role of each is discussed on pages 40–55.

Energy Transfer

To discover how the transfer of ki from the giver of shiatsu to the receiver can be taken to another level, see pages 96–97 on no-touch shiatsu.

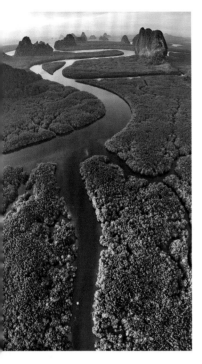

Rivers of energy

The channels through which ki flows have no physical form, although their pathways are precisely defined. They can be likened to rivers running over and through the body.

ENERGY FLOW
Ki flows through the body in channels that form a complex system of links between the organs. There are 12 primary channels that run mainly near the body's surface, named after the organ from which they originate. They are easily manipulated by shiatsu treatment and occur symmetrically on both sides of the body. Extra channels carry ki deeper within the body but only two, the Governing Vessel and the Conception Vessel, are open to shiatsu manipulation.

Channels

The diagrams on this page illustrate the approximate pathways of the 14 channels referred to in this book and the standard abbreviations used. More detailed diagrams of the channels are provided along with the instructions for working on specific areas throughout the book.

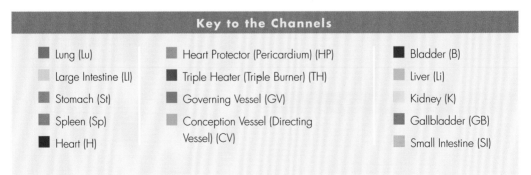

Key to the Channels

Lung (Lu)

Large Intestine (LI)

Stomach (St)

Spleen (Sp)

Heart (H)

Heart Protector (Pericardium) (HP)

Triple Heater (Triple Burner) (TH)

Governing Vessel (GV)

Conception Vessel (Directing Vessel) (CV)

Bladder (B)

Liver (Li)

Kidney (K)

Gallbladder (GB)

Small Intestine (SI)

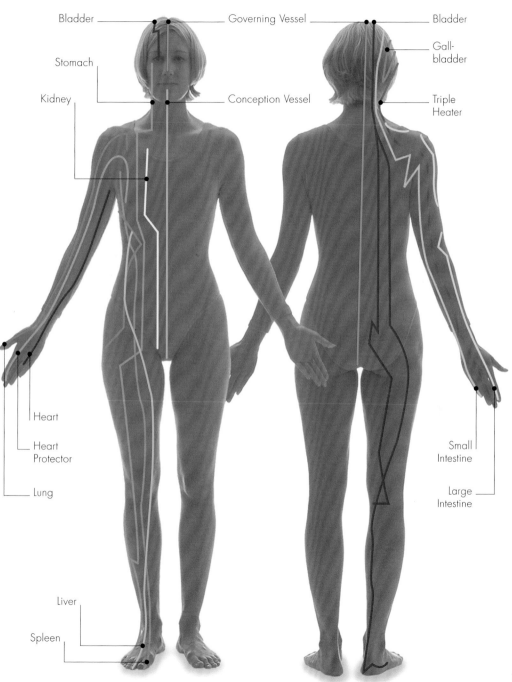

Bladder

Stomach

Kidney

Governing Vessel

Conception Vessel

Bladder

Gall-bladder

Triple Heater

Heart

Heart Protector

Lung

Small Intestine

Large Intestine

Liver

Spleen

Understanding Yin & Yang

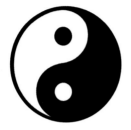

Seeds of change
The taiji *symbol of yin and yang encapsulates the idea that yin is always present in yang and vice versa.*

The theory of yin and yang was first expressed in the ancient *Chinese Book of Changes—the I Ching* (c. 800 BCE). According to this theory, ki, the vital energy that constitutes the "essence" of the universe, comprises two opposing qualities, known as yin and yang. Both aspects are present in different proportions in all things.

Yin/yang symbol

This concept is clearly illustrated in the *taiji*, the yin/yang symbol in which a tiny seed of yin is present within the yang area and vice versa. Although something may be predominantly yin, this state is not immutable. For example, water—a yin substance—has the potential to transform into steam, which is yang. This idea of the potential for change or transformation from yin to yang and yang to yin is fundamental.

Yin/yang body

According to TCM, aspects of the human body and its organs are predominantly either yin or yang. The front of the body is more yin, the back more yang. The front of the body is the site of the yin channels that carry the upward flow of yin energy

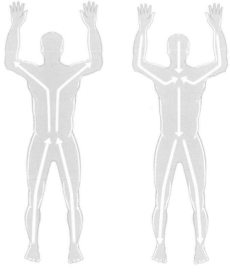

YIN FLOW   YANG FLOW

from the Earth. Yang energy flows from "heaven" through yang channels along the backs of the limbs and the back itself. Yin organs, such as the spleen and liver, tend to be solid and are more concerned with the functions of storage and distribution of energy and blood. Yang organs, such as the Stomach and Bladder, are hollow, and are often concerned with digestion and elimination. See also page 19.

Imbalance or disharmony between yin and yang within the body or within specific organs is thought to underlie many symptoms and the susceptibility to disease. Shiatsu aims to improve well-being by working on the channels through which ki flows to the organs to regulate the balance between yin and yang.

Energy flow

Yang energy flows downward, mainly through channels in the back. Yin energy flows upward, mainly through channels in the front of the body.

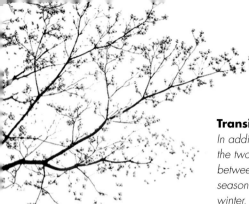

Transitional period

In addition to the simple division between the two states, there is a process of transition between yin and yang. For example, fall, the season in which summer is transformed into winter, is viewed as a time of increasing yin.

YIN & YANG

Yang energy can be characterized as the active force, which carries the impetus for transformation and movement. Yin energy is passive and stabilizing. Both are needed for well-being. A whole system of opposing, but complementary, qualities is based on this understanding and the table on the opposite page provides a selection of major examples. The table also divides the organs according to yin and yang and gives examples of yin and yang foods.

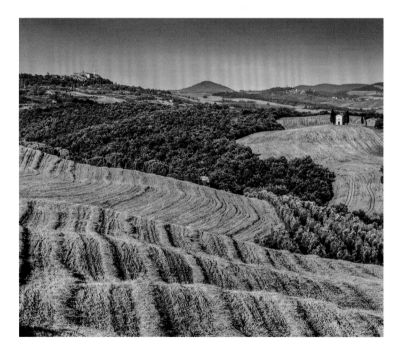

Summer

The characteristics of this season are predominantly yang—long days, heat, evaporating, and dry.

Yang	Yin
KEY CHARACTERISTICS	
Day	Night
Heat	Cold
Summer	Winter
Dry	Wet
Evaporating	Condensing
Ascending	Descending
Active	Still
Exterior	Interior
Heaven	Earth
Male	Female
Immaterial	Material
ORGANS	
Large Intestine	Lungs
Stomach	Spleen
Small Intestine	Heart
Triple Heater	Heart Protector
Gallbladder	Liver
Bladder	Kidneys
FOODS	
Red meat	Lettuce
Garlic	Banana
Peaches	Shellfish
Coffee	Beer
Chili	Tomatoes
Root vegetables	Apples

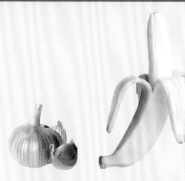

GARLIC   BANANA

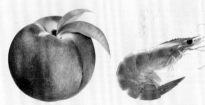

PEACH   SHELLFISH

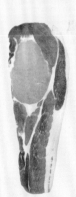

RED MEAT   LETTUCE

Neutral Foods

Rice, nuts, leafy vegetables, wheat, oats, milk, eggs, legumes

The Five Elements

The Five Elements theory developed alongside yin/yang theory and provides further explanation of the way in which ki is manifested in the physical world. Ki occurs in five phases, characterized as Wood, Fire, Earth, Metal, and Water. The theory is a way of understanding how energy transforms from one state to another.

Each element is attributed various characteristics (correspondences) and is believed to govern different aspects of the body and emotions. Both yin and yang qualities occur in each element. The chief correspondences of each element are shown on page 23.

Shiatsu practitioners use the Five Elements theory when analyzing the causes of ill health and to help decide which channels to emphasize during treatment. For information on how this knowledge is applied in relation to specific ailments, see pages 174–215.

Wood
Associated with rising yang (initiation of action), it is characterized by growth and upward movement. When Wood predominates, a person is assertive and organized, but may be prone to anger.

Fire
This represents the peak of yang energy. It embodies emotional warmth and joy, overexcitability, and agitation.

Earth
Defined by increasing yin, this element is associated with ripening and nourishment. Predominance of this element gives a

Five phases of energy
The Five Elements of Earth, Water, Fire, Wood, and Metal represent different qualities of energy and the relationships between those qualities.

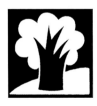

WOOD

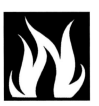

FIRE

EARTH

person the capacity for concentration and listening, which can lead to anxiety and mental anguish.

Metal

Predominantly yin, Metal represents a boundary or point of change. In human terms this is positively characterized by good communication together with a sense of individuality, but, more negatively, sometimes by reserve or withdrawal and defensiveness.

Water

The element of maximum yin, Water always sinks to the deepest place. It stores power and the potential for growth. It can flow with great force and so implies strength of will and self-sufficiency, but may also include fear.

METAL

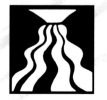

WATER

THE FIVE ELEMENTS IN ACTION

The table of correspondences on the opposite page is intended as a reference. It can be used to expand your understanding of different physical and emotional states viewed according to shiatsu principles. As you become more expert you will get used to observing changes in yourself and others in terms of the Five Elements theory. Practice asking yourself which element is predominant at a particular time.

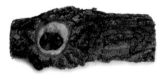

Wood

The Wood element is characterized by the first signs of growth. Wood fuels Fire and stabilizes Earth.

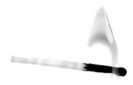

Fire

Emotional warmth and excitability is indicative of the Fire element. Fire enriches Earth and melts Metal.

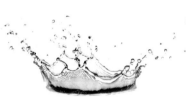

Water

The Water element has the capacity for stillness yet can exert great strength. Water feeds Wood and controls Fire.

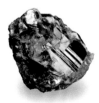

Metal

The Metal element symbolizes a boundary or turning point leading to change. Metal condenses Water and cuts Wood.

Earth

The Earth element is associated with ripening and nourishment. Earth contains Metal and controls the flow of Water.

	WOOD	FIRE	EARTH	METAL	WATER
Direction	East	South	Center	West	North
Season	Spring	Summer	Late summer	Fall	Winter
Cyclic process	Birth	Growth	Ripening	Harvest	Storing
Climate	Wind	Heat	Damp	Dry	Cold
Color	Green	Red	Yellow	White	Blue-black
Flavor	Sour	Bitter	Sweet	Pungent	Salty
Yin organ	Liver	Heart	Spleen	Lungs	Kidney
Yang organ	Gall-bladder	Small Intestine	Stomach	Large Intestine	Bladder
Sense organ	Eyes	Tongue	Mouth	Nose	Ears
Bodily fluid	Tears	Sweat	Saliva	Mucus	Urine
Body tissue	Ligaments and tendons	Blood vessels	Muscles	Skin	Bones
Voice	Shouting	Laughing	Singing	Weeping	Groaning
Emotion	Anger	Joy	Pensiveness	Grief	Fear
Aspect of spirit	Ethereal soul	Mind	Intellect	Corporeal soul	Will

23

Affecting Energy Flow

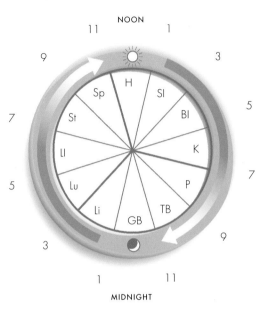

NOON

11   1

9   3

7   5

Sp   H   SI

St   Bl

LI   K

Lu   P

Li   TB

GB

5   7

3   9

1   11

MIDNIGHT

The Chinese clock

The flow of ki is not constant in every part of the body throughout the day, but is said to peak at different times in different channels and organs.

Shiatsu aims to harmonize the flow of ki through the channels that are easily reached from the outside of the body. At a basic level, this is achieved through the application of pressure to specific areas of the body and by "opening" the channels by a variety of stretches and rotations. As you become more expert, you will become better able to sense the subtle energy fluctuations in the person to whom you are giving shiatsu and in your own body. You will also develop a deeper appreciation of the way in which shiatsu allows healing energy to flow between the giver and receiver.

Opening the channels

The energy channels in the body are affected by the state of the muscles and other tissues that surround them. Tense muscles or stiff joints can block the free flow of energy, and the preparatory Makko-ho exercises are designed to counter such blockages. The stretches and rotations that form part of the most basic shiatsu routines also help to open the channels.

Effects of pressure

Ki can be visualized as flowing through the channels in a similar way to water as it flows between the banks of a stream. Along the "stream" are places where the smooth flow is reduced or disrupted. By applying pressure to these areas of deficiency or turbulence, known as *tsubos*, shiatsu is able to influence the flow of ki. Many different parts of the body can be used to apply pressure: thumbs, palms, fingers, elbows, knees, and feet. This book focuses on the use of the hands, because you can control the degree of pressure more easily.

Time
The flow of ki is said to peak at different times in different channels and organs. Some practitioners believe that shiatsu directed at specific channels can be more beneficial if carried out when ki is at its height. However, this is generally not practical. Experienced practitioners take account of the time of day at which symptoms occur in order to assist diagnosis.

Makko-ho Exercises

The preparatory Makko-ho exercises improve the free flow of energy and are useful for both the giver and receiver of shiatsu. These are described on pages 40–55.

WHAT ARE TSUBOS?

Tsubos, or pressure points, are like openings in a channel at which the energy flow can be influenced. Many tsubos occur at specific places along the channels and correspond to points used in acupuncture. They take their names from the channel on which they occur and are numbered in sequence. For example, ʟɪ 4 is the fourth tsubo of the Large Intestine channel. A few tsubos are unrelated to a specific channel.

Locating a tsubo

A tsubo is a point of access to the movement of ki. Pressure on this point can alter the characteristics of the energy flow within the channel.

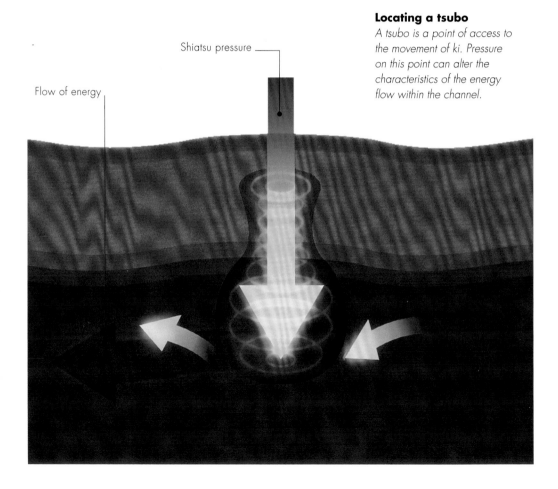

Shiatsu pressure

Flow of energy

Although a tsubo cannot be seen, it can be visualized as a pocket or hollow under the skin. You can be reasonably sure you have located the right place if pressure in the area feels comforting and satisfying to the receiver.

Some tsubos are quite open and relatively large, others are much smaller. Occasionally, there may be discomfort or tenderness when a tsubo is blocked by physical tension. Pressure on a blocked tsubo is best avoided.

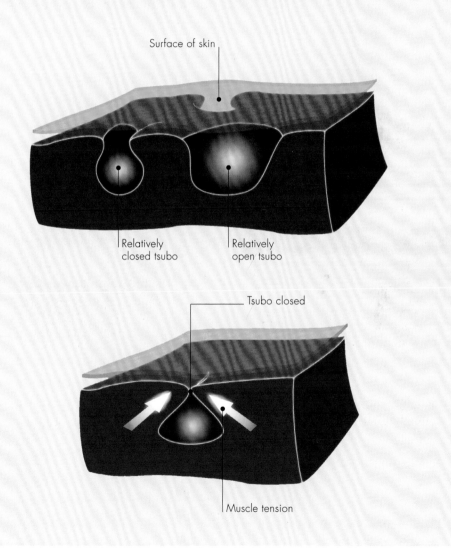

Surface of skin

Relatively closed tsubo

Relatively open tsubo

Tsubo closed

Muscle tension

Energy Need & Fulfillment

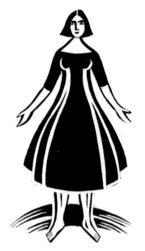

The whole person

Shiatsu takes a holistic approach, treating the whole person, not just the disease, in order to restore well-being.

According to shiatsu, the human body is constantly striving to maintain a balanced energy state. Imbalance may be caused by blockages to the flow of ki within the body or may be the result of external factors, such as temperature changes.

A primary deficiency of energy in a particular channel or tsubo is termed *kyo*. This state of energy "need" provokes a compensatory state of overactivity (known as *jitsu*) elsewhere in that channel or in a related channel in an attempt to restore equilibrium in the body.

Effects

In terms of health and illness, a kyo condition can cause symptoms as a result of the related jitsu response. Various analogies can illustrate this mechanism. For example, lack of food leading to hunger—a kyo state—may lead to an increase in energy expended on the search for food—a jitsu state. The effort spent on searching for food may mean that other tasks are neglected and a succession of adverse consequences may follow. If the basic need for food is fulfilled, the effort put into other activities is restored to normal.

Rebalancing

At any one time there are different areas of kyo and jitsu present within the channels of the body. Sometimes the body can rebalance itself; at other times the imbalance can only be redressed effectively with outside help. Because a kyo state is one of relative "emptiness" or passivity, it is less likely to cause symptoms than the jitsu response it provokes. Jitsu reactions often create tension or pain in the affected tsubo, which is likely to feel "closed" to the giver of shiatsu and pressure should not be applied. It is considered preferable to rebalance by "tonifying"—applying steady pressure to the corresponding kyo tsubo. This encourages the flow of ki to that area, thereby reducing the "need" for the related symptom-causing jitsu reaction. Most basic shiatsu depends on tonifying in areas where ki seems to be insufficient.

Two-handed Connection

Using two hands to create a triangular energy flow is particularly effective for areas of kyo and jitsu—see pages 84–85.

KYO & JITSU DISHARMONY
In a shiatsu session given by an experienced shiatsu practitioner, areas of kyo and jitsu disharmony will be located and adjusted as much as possible. It usually takes time to develop the expertise to identify such areas accurately. Good communication between the giver of shiatsu and the receiver is very important and feedback from the receiver about the effects of the treatment can help you develop your skills.

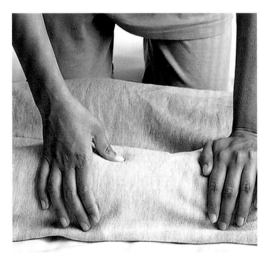

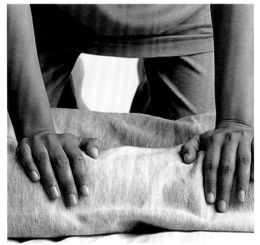

Tonifying
Most basic shiatsu depends on tonifying—that is, strengthening the flow of ki—in areas where it seems to be insufficient. Apply firm, stationary pressure to the tsubo in question. This must be done with sensitivity, without force. The techniques for applying pressure are described on pages 80–97.

Calming
A jitsu tsubo may in some cases respond to calming touch. The best way to do this is to place your palm gently over the area. Contact may either be still or it may be effective to use light, stroking movements. Calming is most likely to be effective if combined with tonifying pressure in a related kyo area.

Dispersal

Although jitsu areas are not normally manipulated by tonifying pressure, in some cases pressure of short duration applied to a tsubo in a jitsu condition can have the effect of dispersing excess energy. This technique is generally most useful when symptoms are of sudden onset (acute). You will also need to apply tonifying pressure to the appropriate kyo area to secure lasting results.

Elbow used to exert insistent, yet gently dispersing pressure to buttock area

Calming touch

Shiatsu & Western Medicine

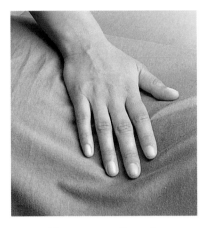

The power of touch

When in pain or distress, people of all cultures recognize the comforting, calming, and healing effect of touch.

Many concepts that underlie shiatsu seem at first glance quite irreconcilable with modern Western medicine, which does not recognize the concept of energy systems. However, an understanding of the effectiveness of human touch is as much part of Western culture as it is of that in the East. We all recognize the healing power of touch—we "rub injuries better" and understand the comforting effect of putting an arm around someone that is in distress or pain. Western high-technology medicine seems to reject the therapeutic value of such instinctive actions, but orthodox medical research is increasingly revealing possible physiological mechanisms to explain the efficacy of therapies such as shiatsu.

Autonomic nervous system

The autonomic nervous system governs the unconscious workings of the body, including processes such as breathing, digestion, and the circulation of blood. It has two divisions, the sympathetic and parasympathetic, which work together to balance the activities of the different organs. The sympathetic nervous system prepares the body for action in the face of perceived danger—the "fight-or-flight" mechanism. The parasympathetic system promotes functions consistent with rest and replenishment of resources.

Effects of shiatsu

Shiatsu seems to have a stimulating effect on the parasympathetic division of the autonomic nervous system, producing an effective counterbalance to the stress-induced tensions that are known to underlie many illnesses and symptoms.

The local effect of shiatsu on painful, tense muscles also finds a basis in modern medical thinking through "pain gate" theories. Pain is transmitted from the site of injury along nerve fibers to the spinal cord and brain. It is possible to block such pain signals if other signals that convey a different sensation, such as pressure, compete with the pain signals for access to the spinal cord, thereby blocking the perception of pain.

Joint Pain

Treatment routines for joint stiffness and pain are detailed pages 188–91.

PREPARING
TO GIVE SHIATSU

Almost everyone is capable of giving and receiving shiatsu; however, be aware of the general cautions described on page 101. Shiatsu is a therapy based on the fundamental human ability to give and receive comfort from physical contact with another. Although many years of study and practice are required to use the technique to its fullest potential, anyone can learn the basics and practice their new skills to good effect on their family and friends. All you need is a basic level of physical fitness and flexibility in order to reach the receiver's body and exert pressure without straining yourself. Most people can benefit from shiatsu treatment, provided that it is carried out with due care.

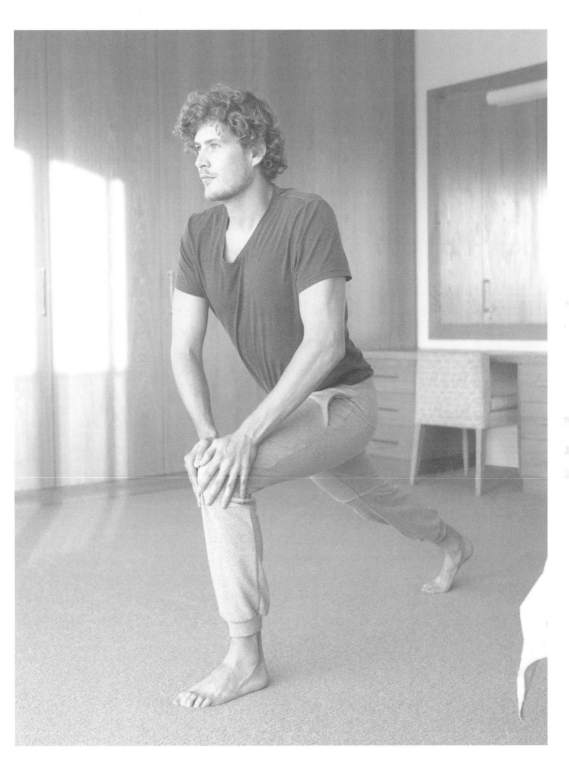

Preparing Mentally

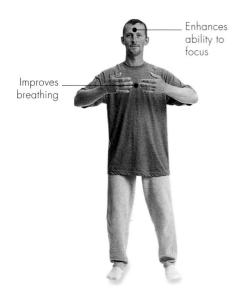

Enhances ability to focus

Improves breathing

Grounding exercises

Enhance the quality of your shiatsu practice through exercise systems such as qigong, which is a form of meditation through movement.

Shiatsu involves giving your full attention and energy to the receiver and to the work you are doing. The treatment cannot be fully effective if your mind is distracted by other thoughts or concerns—your sense of touch will be less attuned to subtle variations in tension and receptiveness in the receiver's body, and your precise control over the degree of pressure will be impaired. Try to cultivate a frame of mind that allows effective verbal and nonverbal communication between both parties.

Meditation

Most people benefit from learning and practicing meditation techniques that enhance mental relaxation and powers of concentration. Different forms of meditation and exercises to promote more effective breathing all have a role in preparing your mind for shiatsu.

Breathing

Breathing is a fundamental vital function. Improved breathing enhances mental focus and increases your physical stamina. As a giver of shiatsu—even a beginner—you need to maximize your mental and physical energies in order to promote better energy flow in those you are treating. A tired and lethargic practitioner cannot give effective treatment. Make the simple breathing exercise on page 39 part of your daily routine.

Mindfulness

An additional mental practice to enhance your shiatsu is to cultivate "mindfulness." This is a way of focusing on the detail of what you are doing at the present moment—even if it is a mundane task such as chopping vegetables. Practice keeping your mind fully absorbed in the task in hand. For example, notice the textures of the vegetables, their colors and their shapes, and the changing pressure exerted on the knife as you peel and slice them.

Keeping your attention focused in this way excludes speculation about the future, remembrance of the past, and any concerns about what is happening elsewhere. It brings you into closer contact with the people and objects around you and develops your powers of observation and capacity for empathy—essential qualities for good shiatsu. The ability to empty your mind completely of any extraneous thoughts and to maintain a chosen focus enhances the sensitivity that you bring to your shiatsu practice.

MENTAL FOCUS TECHNIQUES

Some of the most effective meditation exercises for the beginner involve cultivating breathing awareness. This is particularly valuable for those wishing to perform shiatsu because it helps you become centered on your *hara* (see page 68). Practice meditation daily, if possible, in a quiet room at a time when you will not be disturbed.

Position for meditation

Choose a position in which you feel relaxed and comfortable. This may be cross-legged on the floor, lying down, or seated in a chair. Make sure that the position you select allows you to breathe without restriction.

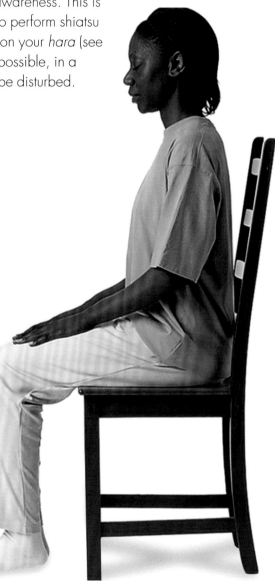

Breathing awareness exercise

1 *Close your eyes and relax. Be aware of your weight sinking into the floor or chair. Feel your limbs getting heavier and your breathing becoming slower, without conscious effort.*

2 *Focus on the sensation of air entering and leaving your nose, without following its passage deeper into the windpipe and lungs. Do this for a few minutes.*

3 *Now change your focus to the sound of your breathing. Notice how the sound of the in-breath is different to that of the out-breath. Continue for a few minutes.*

4 *Shift your focus to the movement of your belly as you breathe. Sense (without looking) how it swells with the in-breath and sinks with the out-breath. Continue for a few minutes before opening your eyes.*

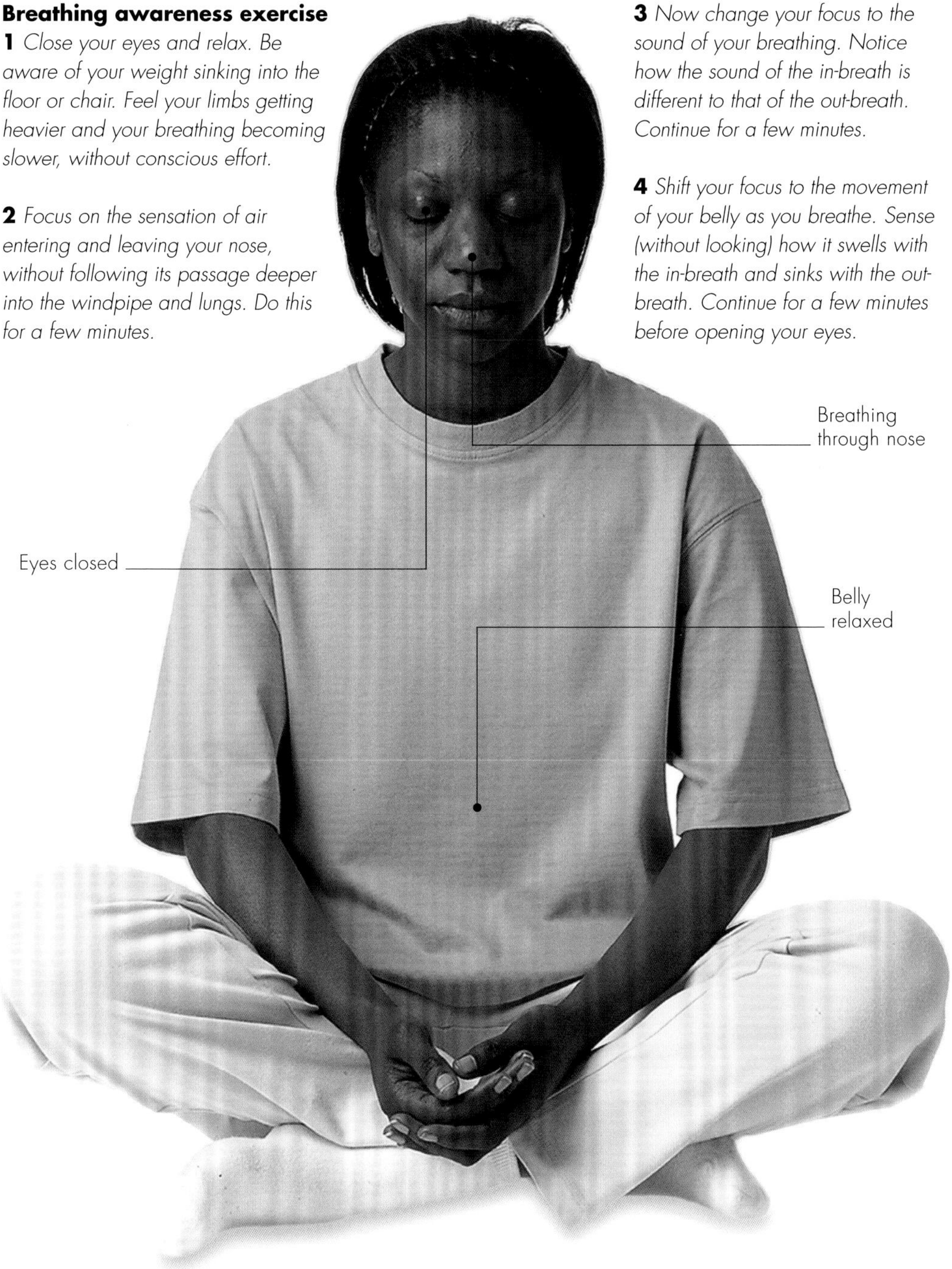

Breathing through nose

Eyes closed

Belly relaxed

Physical Fitness & Makko-ho

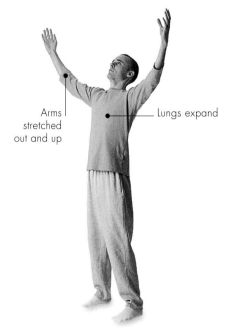

Arms stretched out and up

Lungs expand

Before you start
Stretch the arms upward and outward while breathing in deeply. Relax and lower the arms as you breathe out.

You do not need exceptional physical strength to be able to perform shiatsu effectively, but you do need to be reasonably supple. This helps you avoid straining yourself and ensures that the pressure you apply is always under control so that you do not risk hurting or injuring the receiver.

Makko-ho

Many forms of exercise, especially those arising from Eastern traditions such as yoga, t'ai chi ch'uan, and qigong, can improve your fitness for shiatsu. Makko-ho, the special exercise system devised by Masunaga, the father of modern shiatsu (see pages 8–9), is particularly beneficial. These exercises are intended to improve the flow of ki throughout the body and to maintain flexibility of the joints. These simple, no-strain movements are an excellent form of daily exercise for both givers and receivers of shiatsu. You may like to demonstrate these routines to those you are treating so that they can enhance the benefits of your shiatsu work by practicing between sessions.

Routine

The makko-ho exercises are grouped on the following pages according to the channel they affect. As a daily routine, you can do each exercise described in sequence. In addition, if you identify a ki disharmony in a particular organ or channel and have nobody available to give treatment, opening the relevant channel through the appropriate makko-ho exercises can often bring about an improvement. No special equipment is needed—just wear loose, comfortable clothing. Perform each exercise without straining—do not force any movement that feels uncomfortable. It may take practice to achieve the degree of stretch shown in the photographs.

The first exercise in the sequence (shown on the following page) is for the Lung channel and the Large Intestine channel. The Lung channel governs breathing— the source of vital energy in the body. The Large Intestine channel is associated with respiratory function, as well as with elimination. Disruption of energy flow occurring in either or both of these channels may result from stress and a sedentary lifestyle.

EXERCISES

The accessible, external pathway of the Lung channel extends from just under the collarbone, down the inner arm to the thumb. The Large Intestine channel starts from the index finger and its external pathway runs along the edge of the arm to the shoulder, then up the neck to the nose. The exercise increases the energy flow through both channels. Under no circumstances should you attempt this exercise if you have significant back problems or very low blood pressure.

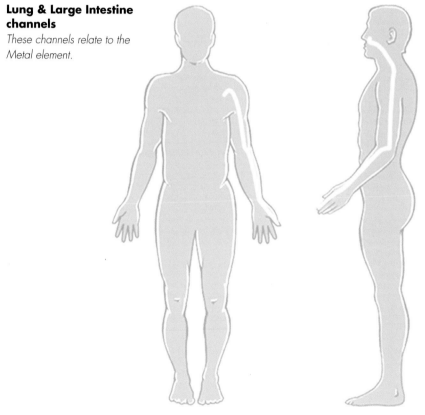

Lung & Large Intestine channels
These channels relate to the Metal element.

LUNG CHANNEL

LARGE INTESTINE CHANNEL

Thumbs linked

Lung makko-ho exercise

Stand with your feet hip-width apart. Link your thumbs behind your back. As you breathe out, lean forward from your hips. Stretch your arms out and keep your knees slightly bent. Take a few breaths and relax into the stretch, allowing your arms to come further over your head if this is comfortable. Straighten up slowly as you breathe out.

Knees slightly bent

Stomach & Spleen

The Stomach and Spleen are related to the Earth element. These organs are associated with obtaining nourishment from food, which increases energy (ki) and blood. In shiatsu theory, blood is the material form of ki and has a vital role in supporting physical growth and the nourishment of all body systems. The latter aspect of this concept accords with the Western view of blood. This nourishing role makes improving energy flow through the Stomach and Spleen channels of special significance in any long-standing illness. Both channels are found on the front of the body.

Stomach channel

The Stomach channel is yang, and therefore the flow of ki through it is downward in direction. A disturbance in the flow of ki can lead to an abnormal upward flow, causing symptoms such as

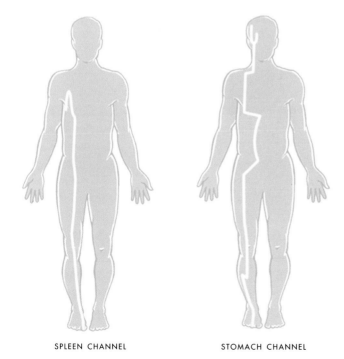

SPLEEN CHANNEL   STOMACH CHANNEL

**Stomach &
spleen channels**
*Both channels are found on
the front of the body and are
related to the Earth element.*

headaches, vomiting, and nausea. The
Stomach channel starts near the nose and
extends into the mouth and up toward the
hairline. From the jaw it continues down
the throat. This lower branch continues
along the collarbone and down the chest
and abdomen. At the groin it takes an
outward path to the front of the thigh and
extends down the front of the leg, ending
on the outside of the second toe.

Spleen channel

The Spleen channel is yin and carries
nourishing grain ki obtained from food
upward to the organs and muscles.
Symptoms of spleen disharmony include
digestive problems, poor appetite,
weakness, and menstrual problems.
The external pathway starts on the inside
edge of the big toe, along the inner
side of the foot and passes up the inside
of the calf and thigh. It enters the lower
abdomen at the groin and re-emerges to
the side of the navel before entering the
abdomen again, where it passes through
the spleen and stomach. Returning to
the surface, it then passes over the ribs
toward the armpit and connects with the
Lung channel under the collarbone.

EXERCISES Perform the following exercises to promote harmonization of the Stomach and Spleen. These exercises are particularly valuable if you have been undertaking intellectual work such as intensive study. The Spleen governs the intellect and can become overstressed in such circumstances, especially if you have also been eating irregularly. Opening the channels can help rebalance your energy, resulting in improved concentration, and may improve stress-related digestive symptoms.

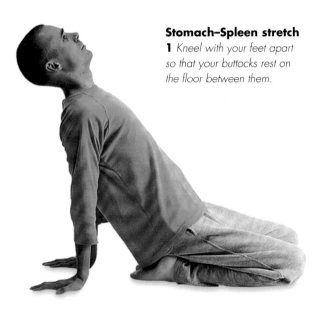

Stomach–Spleen stretch
1 *Kneel with your feet apart so that your buttocks rest on the floor between them.*

2 *As you breathe out, lean back, taking your weight first on your hands and then on your forearms placed flat on the floor. Breathing steadily, relax with your head back and your chest open. If you are supple and you experience no discomfort, drop down further until your back touches the floor. Extend your arms over your head. Breathe in and out three times in your final position before slowly returning to your starting position.*

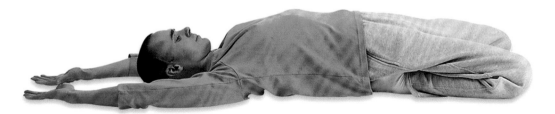

Solar plexus release

Although not part of the original makko-ho program, this is a useful exercise for releasing abdominal tension. Press your fingers into the center of your abdomen under the ribcage. Apply gradually increasing pressure as you lean forward and slowly exhale. Inhale as you come up. Repeat up to five times.

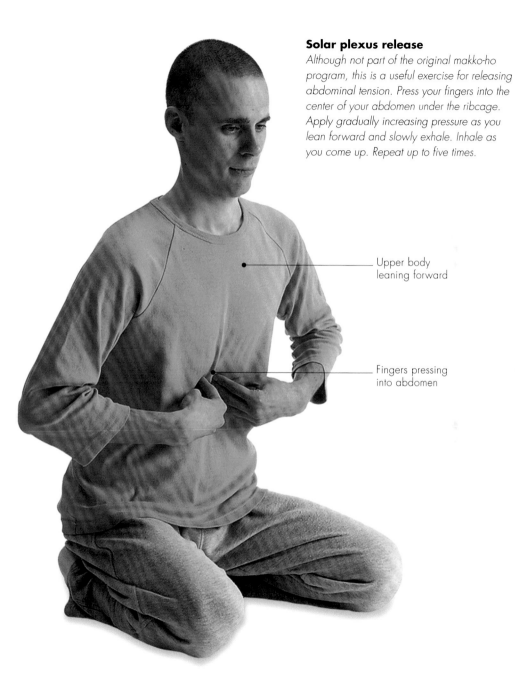

Upper body leaning forward

Fingers pressing into abdomen

Heart, Small Intestine, Bladder & Kidney

The Heart and Small Intestine are related to the Fire element and carry associations of warmth, laughter, joy, and upward movement. Makko-ho exercises for these focus on the front of the body. Those for the Water element organs, the Bladder and Kidney, concentrate on the back.

Organs, channels, & elements

The Heart and Small Intestine are related to Fire, the Bladder and Kidneys to Water.

Heart

Disharmony may manifest as mental restlessness, poor temperature control, or excessive perspiration. Its external path emerges in the armpit and runs inside the arm and palm to the little finger.

Small Intestine

Confused thinking and urinary problems may indicate disturbance of the Small Intestine. The channel travels along the

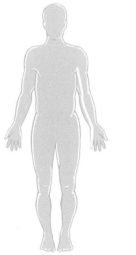

HEART CHANNEL

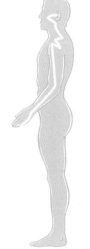

SMALL INTESTINE CHANNEL

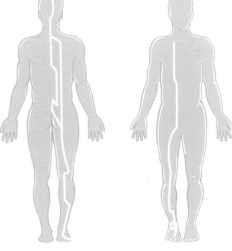

BLADDER CHANNEL   KIDNEY CHANNEL

hand and arm to the shoulder. One branch extends to the ear; the main branch penetrates the chest, linking the Heart, Stomach, and Small Intestine.

Bladder

The Bladder works with the Kidneys and supports the functions of other organs. It also integrates the brain and nervous system. Disharmony is often manifested by restlessness and nervousness. The Bladder channel starts between the eyebrows and extends over the crown of the head, down the spine and legs.

Kidney

The Kidneys are the basis for physical growth and strength, and also rule the bones and hair. Kidney weakness may appear as urinary, reproductive or lower back problems, or general weakness. The Kidney channel originates under the little toe, extends up the inside leg, enters the pelvic cavity, and joins the Conception Vessel in the abdomen.

EXERCISES

Makko-ho exercises for the Heart and Small Intestine and their channels focus on the front of the body. They help to bring a sense of inner calm and concentration. The Bladder and Kidney channels are mainly located in the back and the backs of the legs. These exercises improve energy flow by gently stretching the back, hips, and legs.

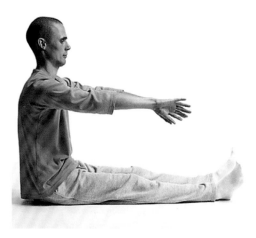 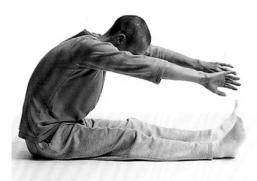

Makko-ho for Bladder & Kidney

1 *Sit on the floor with your legs stretched out in front of you. If you are stiff and find this difficult, it may be helpful to sit on a cushion. Relax your knees and allow your legs to turn outward. Sitting with your weight on the "sitting" bones of the pelvis, breathe in and stretch out your arms, palms outward.*

2 *As you breathe out, bend forward from the hips, keeping your arms and back extended, as if to touch your ankles with your hands. Remain in this position for a few moments, breathing steadily. Let go of tension in your back, neck, shoulders, and limbs.*

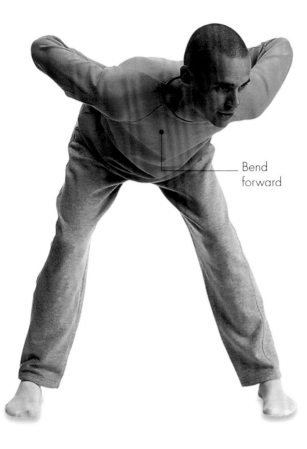

Bend
forward

Rotating from the waist

1 *Although not a part of the original makko-ho program, this additional way of stimulating the flow of ki in the back is very effective. Stand with your feet apart and your hands on your back at waist level.*

2 *Keeping your hips facing forward, rotate your body to one side and bend forward over your knee as you exhale. Circle around until your body is over the other knee, inhale, and lift up. Repeat a few times in alternate directions.*

Makko-ho for Heart & Small Intestine

1 *Sit on the ground with the soles of your feet together. Clasp your feet with your hands and bring them as close to your body as you can with comfort. Breathe deeply.*

2 *As you exhale, bend forward from the hips, bringing your head and chest toward your feet, while keeping your elbows and forearms in front of your shins. Relax in this position, breathing steadily as you focus your attention within the center of your body. Return to the upright position on an "in" breath.*

Heart Protector, Triple Heater, Gallbladder & Liver

Related to the Fire element, the Heart Protector (Pericardium) and Triple Heater (Triple Burner) protect and assist the Heart and Kidneys. The Gallbladder and Liver are organs of the Wood element, implicated in planning, organization, and decisive action.

Organs, channels & elements

The Heart Protector and Triple Heater are related to the Fire element. The Liver and Gallbladder are related to Wood.

Heart Protector & Triple Heater

The Heart Protector defends against heat, infection, and emotional stress. Regulation of this channel may reduce fever and tightness of the chest. It starts in the pericardium, the outer covering of the heart. The Triple Heater harmonizes the workings of the upper, middle, and lower body, and acts as a conduit for energy from the Kidneys to other organs and the body surface. The channel starts at the hand; the main branch ends at the eyebrow.

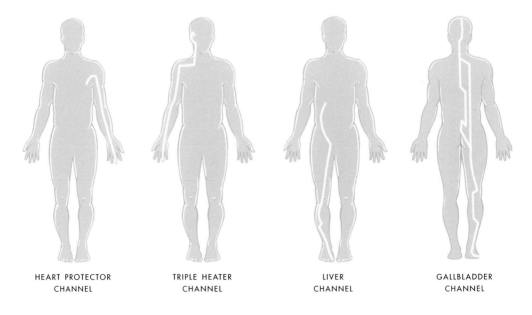

HEART PROTECTOR
CHANNEL

TRIPLE HEATER
CHANNEL

LIVER
CHANNEL

GALLBLADDER
CHANNEL

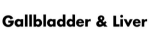

Gallbladder & Liver

Gallbladder blockage may lead to indigestion, headaches, joint stiffness, and indecision. The channel conducts ki from the eye to the base of the skull. It zigzags down the chest and abdomen, enters the pelvic region, emerges behind the hip, and continues down the leg.

The Liver stores blood, the material form of ki, and transports it around the body. Symptoms of liver disharmony include aches and pains, irregularity in body functions, depression, and apathy. The Liver channel starts inside the big toenail. It follows a path over the foot, inside the calf and thigh, and enters the groin. It links the reproductive organs with all other organs. The channel surfaces briefly at the side of the abdomen, but the rest of its pathway is internal.

EXERCISES The makko-ho exercises for these channels improve energy flow by "opening" the sides of the body. The first exercise symbolically reflects the protective role of the Heart Protector and Triple Heater. The Heart Protector channel is enclosed, while the Triple Heater channel is opened to "defend" the body against external threat. The Gallbladder and Liver channels can be opened by side-stretching movements. Side-swinging also helps to move ki through these channels.

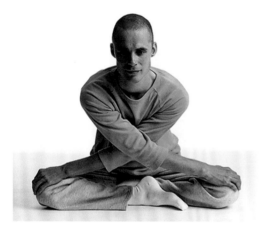

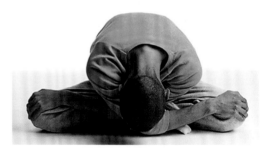

**Makko-ho for Heart Protector
& Triple Heater**
1 *Sit cross-legged, bringing your inside foot as close to the groin as you comfortably can. Cross your arms and clasp each knee with the opposite hand.*

2 *Breathe out and bend forward so that your elbows come down between your knees. Relax your head and neck, allowing them to drop downward. Breathe steadily and come up on an out-breath. Repeat with your arms and legs crossed the other way.*

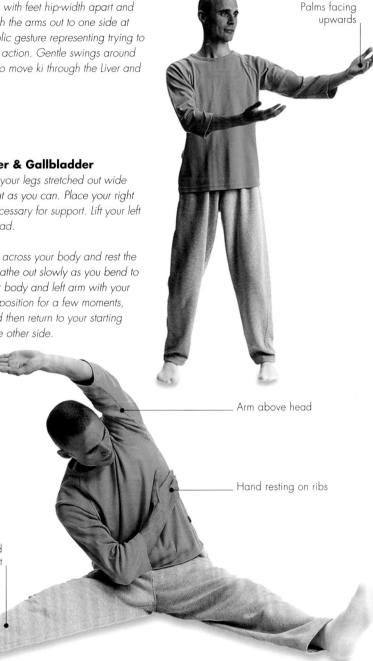

Symbolic stance

The stance of standing with feet hip-width apart and knees slightly bent, with the arms out to one side at waist level, is a symbolic gesture representing trying to decide on a course of action. Gentle swings around to the other side help to move ki through the Liver and Gallbladder channels.

Palms facing upwards

Makko-ho for Liver & Gallbladder

1 Sit on the floor with your legs stretched out wide apart. Sit up as straight as you can. Place your right hand behind you if necessary for support. Lift your left arm up above your head.

2 Bring your right arm across your body and rest the hand on your ribs. Breathe out slowly as you bend to the right, aligning your body and left arm with your right leg. Relax in this position for a few moments, breathing steadily, and then return to your starting position. Repeat on the other side.

Arm above head

Hand resting on ribs

Legs stretched apart

Special Care for Hands & Feet

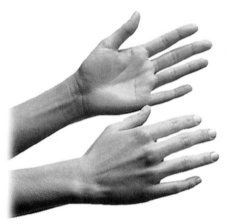

Tools of the trade
Your hands are your essential tools for shiatsu. They need care to maintain their sensitivity.

Your hands are your main tools for giving shiatsu. Fingers, thumbs, palms, and wrists are used to apply pressure to the receiver's body and the quality of the work that you do depends on their condition.

Hands

Hands and fingers need to be strong and supple and sensitive to the variety of signals conveyed by the receiver's body. Aim to eliminate tension, which blocks the flow of ki and reduces your ability to sense subtle differences in the receiver's energy state.

Feet

The feet, too, play an important role in the effectiveness of your shiatsu, mainly through providing a sound grounding. As in other parts of the body, the flow of ki is impaired by muscle tension, so keeping your feet relaxed and supple is essential.

General care

Your hands and feet should be kept clean and well-manicured. It is a matter of respect for the receiver to make sure that your hands are clean and pleasant-looking, so regular maintenance is important. Do not expose your hands to harsh detergents that can inflame and damage the skin. Use a hand or body lotion if your skin has a tendency to roughness. Keep your fingernails short, never allowing the nail to grow longer than the fingertip. This is important because long nails can cause injury when applying fingertip pressure.

Improve energy flow

- Stimulate energy flow in your hands and feet by dipping them in cold water in the morning.
- Walk barefoot whenever safe to do so to provide the muscles and joints of the feet with healthy exercise.
- Shake out your hands regularly during the day, especially after long periods of writing, typing, or other activities that can cause a buildup of tension in the fingers and hands.

Special exercises

The exercises on the following page, called do-in, improve the flexibility and strength of the hands and feet. Take care to work on the left and right sides equally. You may feel an instant improvement in the blood flow through your hands, fingers, feet, and toes.

DO-IN EXERCISES

Practice these exercises daily to maintain suppleness, strength, and optimum sensitivity in your hands and feet. They can be practiced at any time, but take care to work on the left and right sides equally. Even if you do not perform shiatsu every day, you will feel the benefit of these exercises in every manual task you undertake. Start by shaking out your hands to loosen any unconscious tension.

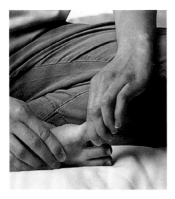 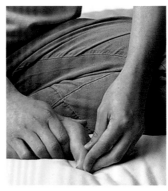 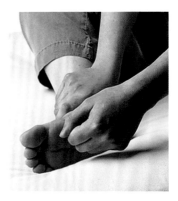

1 *Hold your big toe and rotate it around its knuckle while exerting a gentle pull. Do this in both directions and repeat for each toe on both feet.*

2 *Pull each toe backwards so that you feel a gentle stretch in the underside of the foot. Hold the stretch for a few moments, breathing steadily.*

3 *Use a loosely clenched fist to tap firmly all over the sole of each foot. Enjoy the energizing, tingling feeling in your feet when you stop tapping.*

1 Moving ki from wrist to fingertip

Grip one hand just below the wrist with the other. On an out-breath, squeeze and pull downward from the wrist to the fingertips. Repeat several times on each hand.

Grip just below the wrist

Ki squeezed downward

Fingertips pointing upward

Stretch in heel of hand

2 Wrist-flexing

Place your palms together in front of your chest. Press your hands inward and downward until you feel a stretch in the heel of your hand. Then turn your hands so the fingers are pointing downward and press inward and upward until you feel the stretch.

3 Widening the finger span

Insert the closed fist of one hand into the space between each of your fingers on the other hand, pressing in until you feel a stretch. Do this for both hands.

Stretch between fingers

Press fist between fingers

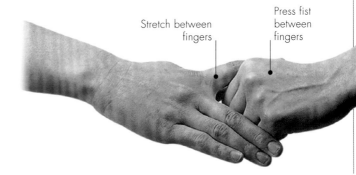

59

General Health Care

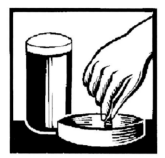

Stay alert
Avoid artificial stimulants and mood-altering substances. Alcohol, coffee, tea, and nicotine fall into this category.

Shiatsu is a process of interaction between the giver and receiver. As a practitioner—even in a modest way—you need to transfer some of your energy via the pressure you apply to the receiver. If your own energy is depleted by illness or, more commonly, by a lack of well-being, your touch will be less effective. It is therefore important for you to take care of your own health. This may mean looking at your lifestyle and eliminating those habits that are likely to deplete your energy and promoting activities that increase your vitality.

Diet

There is no special shiatsu diet, although some people may wish to incorporate ideas of yin and yang into their choice of foods (see page 19). In practical terms, this means ensuring that your diet contains a balance between foods that have yin qualities and those that are more yang. Such ideas are similar to the healthy eating recommendations of Western dieticians, who advise a varied diet in which you should avoid overemphasis on any one group of foods.

Healthy eating

Look to include a high proportion of fresh fruit and vegetables in your diet. These are packed with vitamins and minerals and are easy to digest, providing plenty of energy without a feeling of heaviness. Choose wholegrain cereals over refined products. Wholegrains are digested more slowly and provide a sustained supply of energy. This is preferable to the rapid "energy high" produced by refined carbohydrates, which is followed by a corresponding drop in energy as the blood sugar levels fall. If you are a meateater, do not consume large quantities before a shiatsu session because meat is slow to digest and can lie "heavily" in the stomach, reducing your energy and agility.

Avoid stimulants

Taking any substance that interferes with your natural sensitivity, either in your sense of touch or in your empathy with the person to whom you are giving shiatsu, will reduce your effectiveness. Excessive amounts of caffeine, prescription tranquilizers, alcohol, and other mood-altering drugs, can have this effect on your natural sensitivity.

Yin & Yang

Yin foods include bananas, shellfish, tomatoes, and beer, while foods such as red meat, garlic, and coffee are very yang. See page 19 for more details.

SHIATSU CLOTHING

The practice of shiatsu requires no specialized clothing but both giver and receiver should be warm and comfortable, and have freedom of movement. The receiver is not required to remove any clothing other than shoes—pressure is applied through the fabric of the garments and this does not in any way impair its effectiveness. Both parties may find a loose T-shirt with pajama-style trousers or thin jogging pants a good solution.

Go natural

For both parties, light, natural fabrics are preferable because their texture seems to allow more effective transmission of sensation.

Cotton is a good fabric

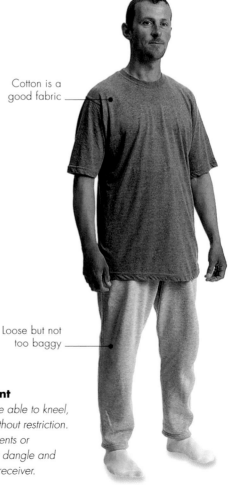

Loose but not too baggy

Ease of movement

The giver needs to be able to kneel, bend, and stretch without restriction. Avoid wearing garments or accessories that may dangle and distract you and the receiver.

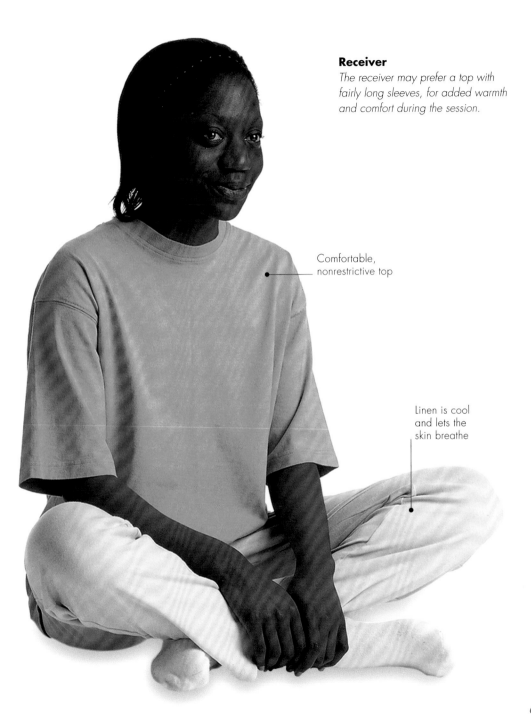

Receiver

The receiver may prefer a top with fairly long sleeves, for added warmth and comfort during the session.

Comfortable, nonrestrictive top

Linen is cool and lets the skin breathe

The Shiatsu Environment

The room in which you give shiatsu should be conducive to the sense of harmony and tranquility you aim to encourage in the receiver. Try to reserve a space exclusively for the practice of shiatsu. You will need enough floor space for the receiver to lie down and for you to move around without being cramped.

Lighting

Natural lighting and good ventilation are important. If you are doing shiatsu after dark, choose soft artificial lighting rather than harsh fluorescent lights. The room should be warm, but not too hot.

Furniture

Remove as much unnecessary furniture and clutter as possible. This will help you and the person you are treating to concentrate on the shiatsu and its effects.

Scents & sounds

Some practitioners like to scent the room with essential oils using an aromatherapy

Tranquil surroundings

An ideal shiatsu area provides few distractions and plenty of space for you to move around.

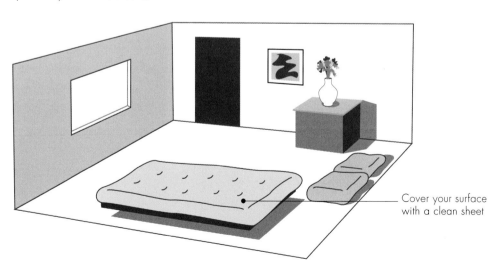

Cover your surface with a clean sheet

vaporizer. This is a matter of personal preference, but if you decide to do this, select your oil with care—an intrusive scent may detract from the treatment. In a similar way, some people like to play music during a shiatsu session. This can be relaxing if it is not too loud and if the choice of music is acceptable to both.

Lying down area

The main item of equipment you need is a suitable surface for the receiver to lie down on. A thin futon is ideal, soft enough for the receiver's comfort but sufficiently firm to allow you to apply effective pressure. You can improvize by folding several blankets to provide a generous layer of padding. Cover your surface with a clean sheet.

You will also need a small, thin cushion to support the receiver's head and a selection of pillows to provide additional support in certain positions. It may also be useful to have a light cotton blanket available. You can use this to cover the parts of the receiver's body that are not being worked on in order to provide a continuing sense of warmth and security.

BASIC SHIATSU TECHNIQUES

Any would-be giver of shiatsu should expect to spend some time learning basic shiatsu techniques before any serious attempt to treat another person. Ideally, you should join a class where an experienced teacher can demonstrate the correct way of giving shiatsu and observe and comment on your own developing skill. However, this chapter aims to provide a useful introduction to the techniques of good shiatsu. A shiatsu session with a well-qualified practitioner is strongly recommended—only by experiencing the different sensations that result from shiatsu pressure and stretches can you truly empathize with the feelings of those who will be receivers of your shiatsu.

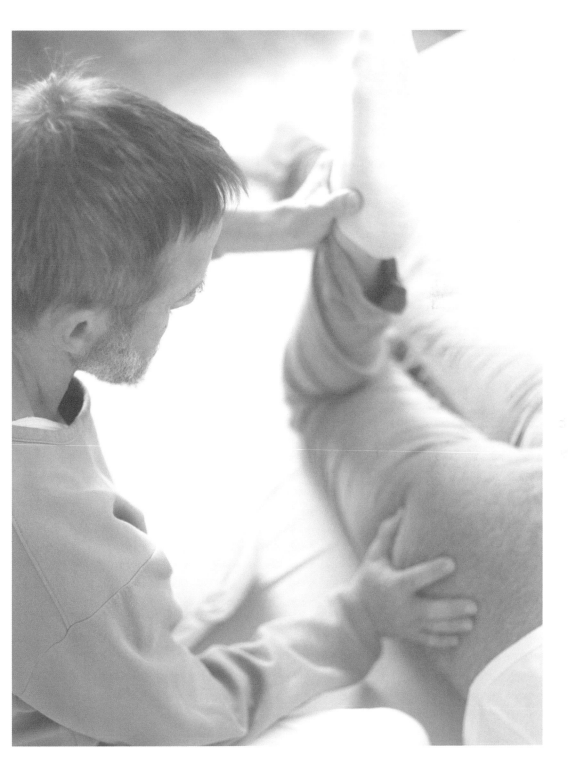

Using Weight & Gravity

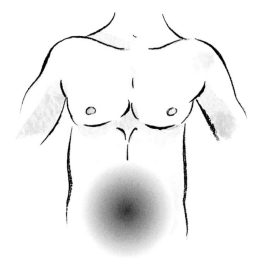

Tanden & hara

Your hara, or center of gravity, surrounds your tanden, which is three finger-widths below your navel.

The essence of shiatsu is the use of pressure without force. The key to appreciating the difference is an understanding of the role of your center of gravity—called the *hara* in Japanese.

Location

The hara is located in your abdomen around a central point about three finger-widths below the navel, known as the *tanden*. The hara is not only the pivotal point of your body in terms of weight distribution, it is also the center of its "life force." Movement or pressure directed from this center is backed up by the weight and vitality of the body and requires less exertion. In shiatsu you always aim to utilize energy from the hara in order to apply pressure, not simply the muscular strength of the limb you are using.

Awareness

The concept of hara also encompasses your emotional and psychological well-being. Focusing on your inner center helps to harmonize body, mind, and spirit. It can help build a sense of self-confidence and purpose. When you practice shiatsu with hara awareness, you are developing your internal resources and this will affect other aspects of your life. You also enhance your capacity to transmit healing energy to others.

Identification

First identify your hara and tanden. In an easy sitting position with your legs comfortably apart, put your hand over your tanden three finger-widths below your navel. Relax your stomach muscles so that your abdomen is distended, close your eyes and breathe steadily. With your eyes closed, turn your gaze down toward this inner center of your being and try to get a sense of the energy gathered in the surrounding area of your abdomen. You can then proceed to the hara awareness exercises on the following pages, which are intended to help you develop an understanding of your hara and the ways in which you can utilize your inner energy when you practice shiatsu.

Inner Energy

If your hara is strong, you are better able to withstand life's disappointments and setbacks. You are focused on your own goals and do not waste your energy or talents.

HARA AWARENESS

Having gained a sense of the location and energetic qualities of your hara, try these exercises to alter your weight distribution and direct pressure through your limbs. Moving around the floor on all fours is unfamiliar to most adults, but it is an essential part of shiatsu, in which all treatment is given at floor level. You need to regain the sense of contact with the ground that you had as a crawling baby.

1 *Gain awareness of your hara by a simple breathing exercise. In a comfortable sitting position, place both your hands on your lower abdomen. With your stomach muscles relaxed, breathe in through your nose so that your belly distends. As you breathe out through your nose, your belly will contract. Feel the energy gathering in your belly with each in-breath.*

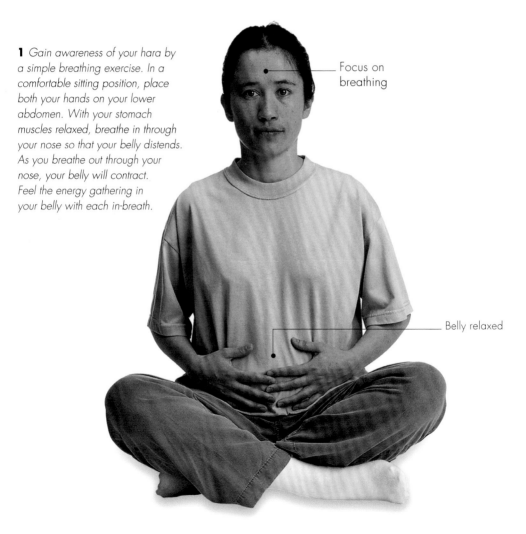

Focus on breathing

Belly relaxed

2 *Kneel on the floor with your legs apart and place your hands wide apart in front of you. Start by having all your weight on your knees. Gradually move your body forward so that your hands and arms begin to take more of your weight (try to visualize this as a movement of the hara). Pause when you sense that your weight is evenly distributed between your limbs.*

3 *Move your hara in a circle and notice how your weight transfers between your limbs as your center of gravity shifts. Practice shifting more weight onto the limb of your choice and notice how the weight carried by the remaining limbs is redistributed.*

The Importance of Stance

The standard shiatsu stances are based on kneeling or squatting. These positions (see pages 74–75) provide a stable base for floor work and permit a range of movement around the receiver. Most adults in Western societies do not find it easy to sit and work in these positions without practice. However, it is worth retraining your body for these ways of sitting since they generally place less strain on the back than sitting on chairs. Sit in the following positions at any time you can: when watching television or reading, or when playing on the floor with small children.

Kneeling in seiza

The standard kneeling position, with the feet tucked under the buttocks, is known in Japanese as *seiza*. You can do much shiatsu from this position because it provides a firm base and allows you to reach forward when necessary.

Knees wide

A variation on seiza is with the knees spread wide. Take care not to sit too close to the person's head with your knees spread apart. This can be offensive and threatening; do not allow your knees to extend beyond their ears.

Comfortable & effective
Shiatsu is most effective when both giver and receiver are in a comfortable position. Strain or tension can block the flow of energy.

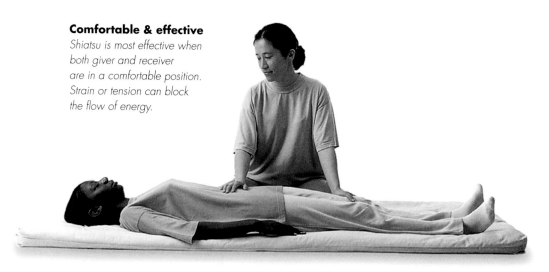

Half-kneeling

You will sometimes need to use this
position for stretching and manipulating
the limbs. The bent knee can be used
to support a part of the body you are
working on.

Squatting

Most Westerners will find they are not
sufficiently stable in this position to work
in it for more than a few minutes at a time.
But practicing the squat can be very
beneficial for flexibility.

Half-squat

Holding a position between squatting
and kneeling lets you sit a little taller than
in seiza and allows you to move sideways
as you work. It provides an effective
position for directing hara energy around
the body.

Japanese Tradition

Kneeling in seiza is the position in which
Japanese people traditionally sit for meals at low
tables. It is also used for the Tea Ceremony and
for meditation.

STANCE VARIATIONS

You can use a variety of positions based on kneeling or squatting for giving shiatsu. Much depends on what you find comfortable—adults in Western societies may find some of these positions difficult. The choice of position is also affected by the area being treated and how far across the body you need to reach. You will also need to consider how the position you choose affects the alignment of your hara (see page 78).

Kneeling in seiza
Kneel with your knees together. Rest your buttocks on your heels with your insteps flat on the floor. You can adapt this position to the knees-wide stance.

Half-kneeling
From seiza, raise one knee and place the foot flat on the ground to the side.

Half-squat
From the half-kneeling position, raise the lower knee so that the foot is resting on the toes.

Seiza alternative
As for the standard seiza kneeling position, but with your feet resting on the toes.

Squatting
With your feet placed wide apart, lower your body toward the ground. Lean forward between your knees for stability.

Avoiding Strain

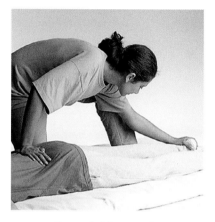

Potential for strain
*Positions in which you stretch over
the receiver in order to exert pressure
are most likely to lead to strain.*

A good shiatsu practitioner is always aware of how their practice of shiatsu affects themselves as well as the receiver. Strain or tension can block your energy, resulting in ineffective shiatsu. Many people find regular practice of yoga or t'ai chi ch'uan, for example, helps them to develop an innate sense of how to use the body in a sensitive and balanced way. Applying a few key principles as you work will help protect yourself from strain and possible injury.

Relax

Keep your whole body relaxed. Look for signs of tension such as hunched shoulders and shallow breathing.

- Keep your neck lengthened and let your shoulders relax downward.
- Open your chest and relax your abdomen as you breathe deeply.
- Keep your gaze ahead. Avoid looking down at your hands once they are correctly positioned.
- Visualize all your joints loosening and opening.

Weight underside

Focus on keeping your weight "underside." This is a concept that implies a division of the body into upper and lower aspects. The lower aspects, such as the undersides of the arms or legs as you kneel on the ground, receive energy from the ground and feel heavier than the ungrounded, upper aspects. Movement should be directed from these lower aspects to the upper parts.

Wide base

Select a working position in which your weight is distributed over as wide an area as possible. Stances in which the knees are widely spaced are generally preferable, especially when there is a need to apply strong pressure. They provide better balance and therefore better control, and they increase the "underside" areas. Such stances also open your hara.

Back protection

Position yourself so pressure is distributed ·evenly along the spine so that no single area is overstressed.

- Get as close to the area on which you are working as possible.
- Keep your back straight, but not rigid, as you work, and avoid curving or arching your spine.

Back & Shoulder Work

Sitting positions for back and shoulder work on people who find lying down inconvenient or difficult are shown on pages 164–71.

ALIGNING YOUR HARA

When you position yourself next to the person you are treating, ready to start work, always bear in mind the need to keep your hara open—that is, keep your limbs and chest spread wide. As you move around to treat different areas, consider how to align your hara with the area on which you are working. Aim to adopt a position in which your abdomen is facing the area you are about to treat.

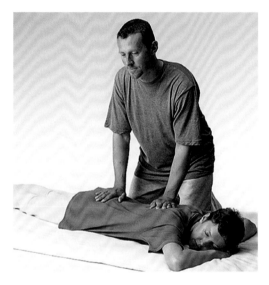 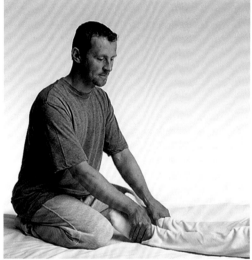

Working from the side

In this position, the knees-wide stance of the shiatsu giver, at 90° to the receiver's back, allows optimum use of hara energy.

Working at the feet

By straddling the recipient's feet, the giver effectively directs hara energy toward the lower leg area where he is working.

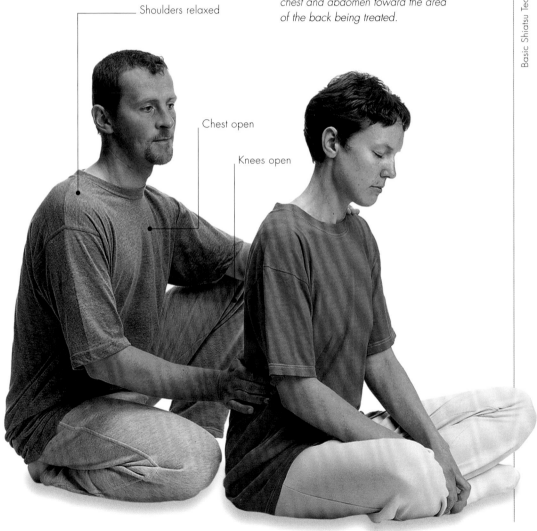

Working in a sitting position
The giver adopts a relaxed, half-kneeling position, which opens his chest and abdomen toward the area of the back being treated.

Shoulders relaxed

Chest open

Knees open

Hand & Arm Contact

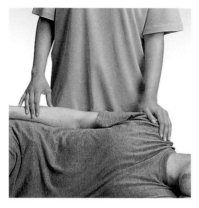

Energy flow

When the giver of shiatsu relaxes her shoulders, arms, and hands, there is an effective flow of energy to the receiver.

Your arms and hands are the principal means through which you will be giving shiatsu. You can apply pressure with the palms, fingers, thumbs, and elbows, depending on the size of the area to be treated and the quality of touch you want to administer. Finger and thumb pressure is discussed on page 88; use of the elbows is described on page 92.

Palm pressure

Working with the palm is perhaps the best technique with which to start. Many shiatsu sessions begin with the giver sitting "in hara"—that is, comfortable, centered, and relaxed—with their palm in contact with the receiver's hara. The palm provides a reassuring pressure for the receiver and is a sensitive monitor of the receiver's energy state for the giver. During treatment, palm contact is both supportive and "tonifying"—a shiatsu term that means stimulating to the flow of ki. Palming can vary from gentle touch to firm, penetrating pressure.

Position

Position yourself so that your arm is at a right angle to the surface of the area to be treated. Keep your arms fairly straight, but relaxed. Tense joints block the flow of energy and reduce your sensitivity to the receiver's response. Keep the whole of your palm in contact with the receiver's body, molding it to the shape of the body part being treated.

The palms are best suited to the application of stationary pressure: pressure applied steadily, without movement or variation. Lean into your palm but, as you apply pressure, be aware of signs of response from the receiver and stop if treatment is painful or uncomfortable.

Hand heel

In some cases, if you want to focus treatment on a smaller area, for example, it is possible to emphasize contact through the heel of the hand instead of using the whole palm. Place the heel of the hand over that area, allowing the palm to rest gently in contact with the adjacent area. Use subtle adjustments of your center of gravity to direct your weight into the heel of your hand.

Dragon's Mouth

This technique applies pressure using the area between the thumb and index finger. The main contact is made with the knuckle bone at the base of the index finger. This method is useful for work on curved areas such as arms or the base of the skull.

USING HANDS & ARMS

The hand contains important energy centers which shiatsu practitioners exploit. An important tsubo of the Heart Protector channel—HP 8 or *laogong* – is located in the center of the palm under the joint of the third finger. The energy carried by the Heart Protector has a reassuring and healing quality. It is also associated with joy and communication. With practice, you can transmit some of these feelings when you give shiatsu.

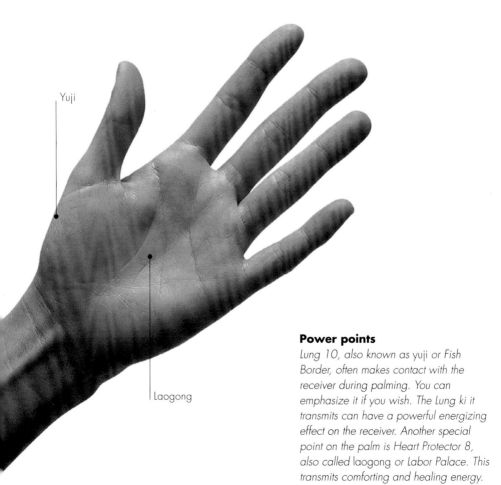

Yuji

Laogong

Power points

Lung 10, also known as yuji or Fish Border, often makes contact with the receiver during palming. You can emphasize it if you wish. The Lung ki it transmits can have a powerful energizing effect on the receiver. Another special point on the palm is Heart Protector 8, also called laogong *or Labor Palace. This transmits comforting and healing energy.*

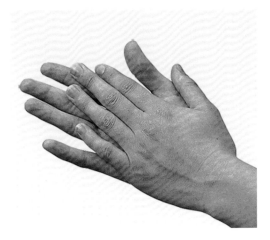

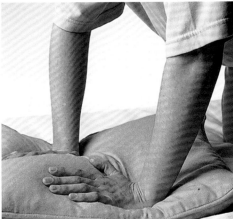

Preparing your hands
A brisk rub of your palms before you make contact with the receiver maximizes the flow of ki.

Practice exerting pressure
Practice on a cushion. Use your weight, not strength, and keep your elbows slightly bent.

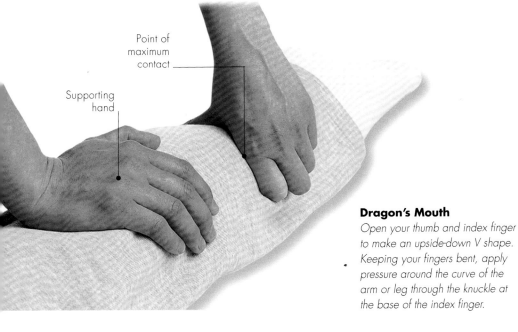

Point of maximum contact

Supporting hand

Dragon's Mouth
Open your thumb and index finger to make an upside-down V shape. Keeping your fingers bent, apply pressure around the curve of the arm or leg through the knuckle at the base of the index finger.

83

The Supporting Hand

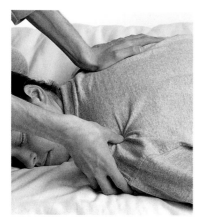

Both hands at work
The lower active hand thumbs the tsubo, while the upper passive hand provides support.

When you perform shiatsu, you usually use one hand to apply pressure (except on some occasions when a two-handed technique may be more appropriate). The less active hand nevertheless has an important supporting function in your treatment. On a philosophical level, shiatsu theory is based on the interplay of the complementary qualities of yin and yang, passive and active. The active use of one hand and the passive presence of the other hand impart a harmonious unity to the shiatsu treatment. While the active hand instigates changes in the flow of energy in the receiver's body, the support hand "listens" to his or her response to that stimulus. The placement of two hands on the receiver's body deepens and extends the benefits of treatment.

Energy triangle

The two-handed connection creates a triangular energy flow between your hara and the active and passive hands, with the area of the receiver's body between the two hands forming one side of the triangle. This energy circuit has a particular significance when dealing with areas of kyo and jitsu (see pages 28–31). Keep the passive hand in gentle contact with a jitsu area on a particular channel while using the active hand to apply stationary pressure to a kyo area on that channel. With developing sensitivity, you may be able to detect energy gathering in the kyo area and dispersing in the jitsu area. The result is a successfully rebalanced energy flow.

Support

The passive hand can also perform an important practical supporting role. When you want to apply pressure to a part of the body that is not resting on the floor, you can use the passive hand to support that part while you apply pressure with the other hand. Such support creates a sense of security for the receiver, as well as providing the necessary resistance to the pressure.

Maintain contact

Always keep one hand in contact with the receiver's body. If both hands are removed for more than a moment or two, the communication between giver and receiver is severed and you are likely to have to spend time re-establishing it. Plan sessions so that you work on the receiver in an order that allows you to leave one hand in contact as you move into each new position.

SUPPORTING MOVEMENTS
You can practice ways of coordinating the use of both hands. There are no strict rules for this, but as a general guideline the passive hand should be placed on the part of the channel nearest the center of the body, while the active hand works on the more distant parts of the same channel. Remember that the same hand does not always have to be the active one.

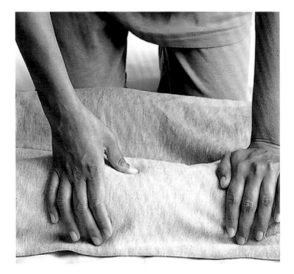

Energetic support

In this photograph the hand on the left is the active hand, applying thumb pressure to a channel in the leg. The hand on the right is the passive hand, monitoring the receiver's response.

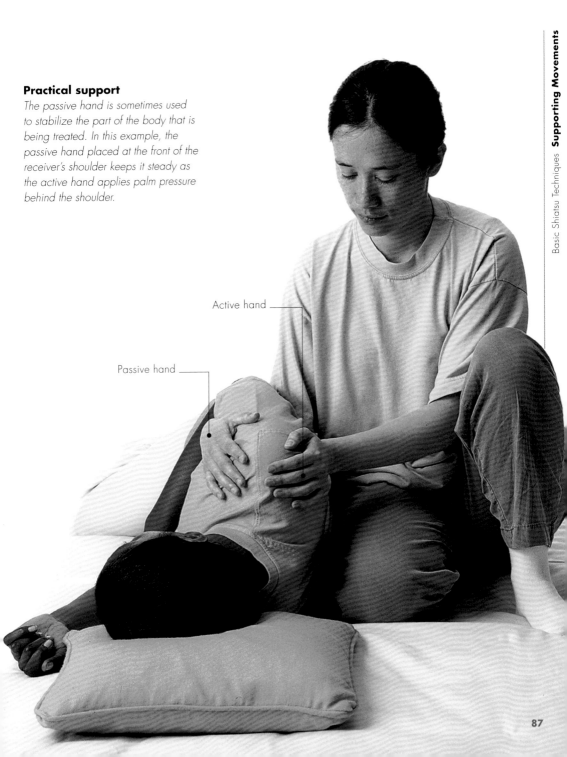

Practical support

The passive hand is sometimes used to stabilize the part of the body that is being treated. In this example, the passive hand placed at the front of the receiver's shoulder keeps it steady as the active hand applies palm pressure behind the shoulder.

Active hand

Passive hand

Thumb & Finger Action

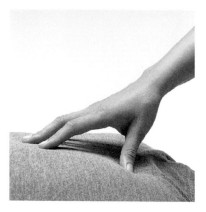

Thumb pressure
This shows correct use of the thumb as an extension of the arm, comfortably supported by the fingers of the same hand.

While the palms are excellent for giving generalized shiatsu along the channels, the smaller dimensions of the fingers and thumbs make them better tools for applying concentrated pressure to specific tsubos. A tsubo is said to be about the same size as the thumb tip.

Thumb

This is the strongest digit and is used to apply deep, penetrating pressure in most areas of the body. The result is greater stimulation of ki than with the more dispersed pressure from the palms. This type of pressure is also useful for alleviating knots of tension in areas of muscle. Place the extended thumb at a right angle to the area being treated, with the flat surface of the thumbtip in contact with the receiver. Use your weight to apply stationary pressure through your arm, hand, and thumb. The thumb joint may bend back a little as you do this. If this happens to a significant degree, consider using an alternative means of applying local pressure such as the finger joint. Never allow your thumb joint to "hook" inward (see page 91). This blocks the flow of energy and may cause discomfort to the receiver. Use your splayed fingers to balance and support the thumb.

Fingers

The fingers can also be used to give shiatsu in localized areas. They are suitable for fine work on the head and face, where the greater force of thumb work is not suitable. The fingers of both hands can be used simultaneously along the same channels on each side of the body, for example, along the Bladder channel on either side of the spine. A variety of finger techniques are used. Often the index and third fingers are used together, which provides greater stability under pressure. The section of the index finger between the first and second joints can also be used for administering local pressure, usually in conjunction with the thumb of the same hand.

Practice

You can practice thumb and finger work on a firm cushion or on an upholstered piece of furniture. While you are practicing, check that your joints are not strained by the application of excessive force. When you work on a real person, increase pressure through your thumbs and fingers only gradually. Concentrated pressure of this type can cause pain—relax your pressure and moderate your technique if this occurs.

THUMBS & FINGERS
Your thumbs and fingers are the precision tools of shiatsu. Use them to treat individual tsubos. Your thumbs are strong enough to support a considerable degree of pressure, although this is unlikely to be needed. The fingers are particularly useful in situations where precise and sensitive pressure is required, such as when treating the face. There are many ways of using your thumbs and fingers, of which only a selection are shown here. When you have mastered the basic principles, you may decide to experiment with your own techniques.

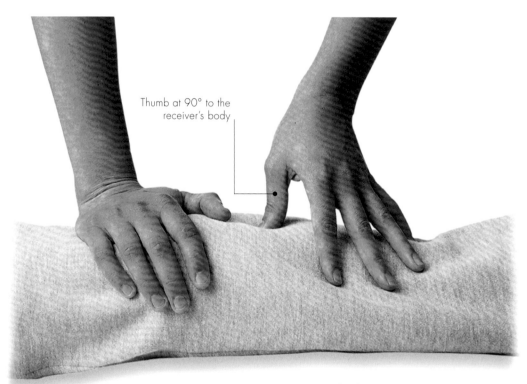

Thumb at 90° to the receiver's body

How to apply thumb pressure
Make contact with the flat of the thumb-tip and splay the fingers for support. Use your body weight and your center of gravity to create and direct the pressure.

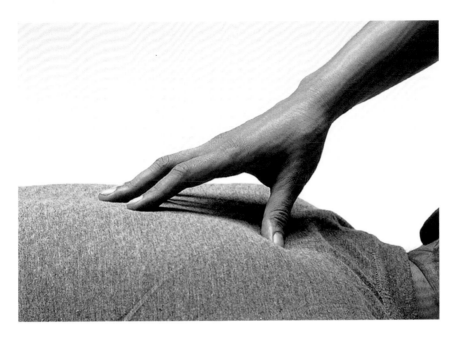

Good technique
This shows the correct use of the thumb as an extension of the arm comfortably supported by the fingers of the same hand.

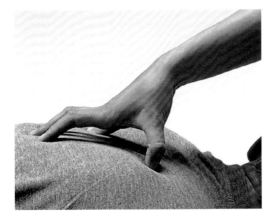

Bad technique
This clearly shows faulty technique—the fingers are tense and the thumbs are hooked, so the flow of energy will be blocked.

Elbow, Knee & Foot Pressure

Shiatsu is a therapy that involves the whole body of both the giver and receiver. Our hands and arms are our main "tools" but there will be times when the use of another part of the body will be the perfect solution.

Elbows

The elbows play a key role in shiatsu. The way you use your elbows can affect the energy flow in your arms and hands. They can also be used to apply pressure in areas where a stronger action is required. Elbow pressure is ideal for dispersing tension in well-muscled parts

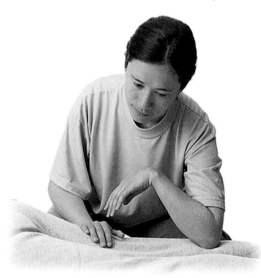

of the body, such as the buttocks, hips, shoulders, and thighs, but it may be too forceful for those with a fragile physique. Use your fingers to identify the area needing treatment before applying the underside, not the point, of the elbow to that area. Gently lean into the elbow, gradually increasing the weight applied if it is acceptable to the receiver.

Knees

The knees are suitable for applying pressure to the backs of the thighs or to the lower back when the receiver is in a sitting position. Knee pressure should be used by novice shiatsu practitioners with great caution and only on those of reasonably robust physique. You need to be confident that you can control the degree of pressure exerted so that you do not cause pain or injury. Use your hands for balance and support as you shift your weight onto the knee.

Elbow power
The elbows are able to provide blunt pressure that is ideal for releasing tension in large muscles, such as those of the leg.

Feet

Your feet carry your entire body weight
and can be used to apply strong
pressure. The beginner should only use
the feet for working on the undersides
of the receiver's feet, which are equally
designed to withstand the weight of a
whole body. While the receiver is prone
(lying on her stomach), stand with your
heels on the ground and the balls of your
feet in the arch of the receiver's feet. The
contours of your soles should fit neatly into
those of the receiver. Gradually shift your
weight forward from your heels onto the
balls of your feet and thereby onto those
of the receiver. Be prepared to release the
pressure if the receiver finds it too forceful.

ELBOWS, KNEES & FEET
Other parts of your body may be used when your hands need a rest, or if they seem better suited to treat the required area. Practice using the elbows, knees, and feet as shown. Pressure given using these parts of the body can be greater than that given by the hands, so listen for feedback—both verbal and in the form of altered sensation—from the receiver and adjust treatment as necessary.

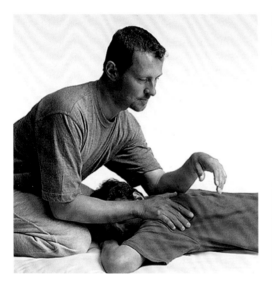

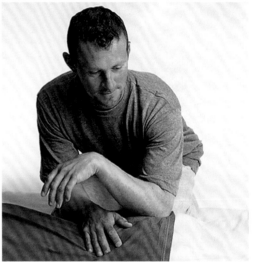

Elbow to shoulder
Use the flat underside of the elbow, not the point, to apply strong pressure to tense muscles in the shoulder. Direct your weight by shifting your center of gravity. Use your other hand for continuing support and connection, and to sense changes in the receiver's response.

Elbow to buttocks
The large muscles of the buttocks benefit from strong treatment that can be given through the underside of the elbow. Position yourself so that your arm is more or less perpendicular to the buttock area. Gradually shift your weight forward to provide pressure.

Feet to feet

With the receiver lying prone, stand on his feet so that the balls of your feet fit into the arch of his feet. Keep your heels on the ground. Gradually move your center of gravity forward so that your weight slowly shifts onto the balls of your feet and exerts pressure on the receiver's.

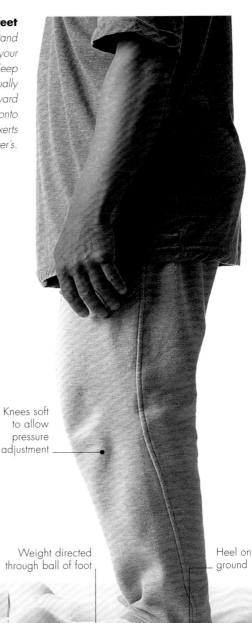

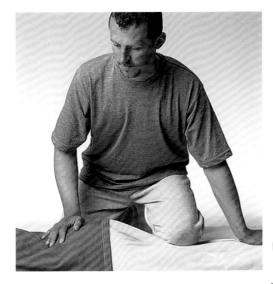

Knees soft to allow pressure adjustment

Knee to thigh

Start from a stable kneeling position, balanced by your hands. Place your knee on the back of the receiver's thigh, without applying force. Then slowly shift your weight forward so that the pressure on the thigh gradually increases. Do not apply pressure beyond the point of comfort for the receiver.

Weight directed through ball of foot

Heel on ground

No-touch Shiatsu

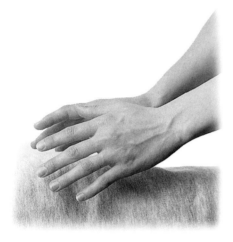

Energy transfer
Some practitioners are able to transmit healing energy simply by holding their hands over the area to be treated.

M uch has already been said about the importance of the transfer of energy, or ki, between the giver and receiver of shiatsu. This invisible and unquantifiable exchange makes shiatsu much more than a pleasant form of bodywork. The means by which energy is transferred are subtle and to some extent inexplicable. We can really only judge what occurs by asking the receiver what he felt during the treatment— did he feel better and, if so, in what ways?

Certain benefits can be gained from the basic physiological effects of the application of pressure to different areas of the body. But a good shiatsu practitioner who has developed his knowledge, sensitivity, and powers of observation to a high degree will always provide more effective treatment than a practitioner with lesser skills.

Minimum contact

Some practitioners have taken their practice to such a degree of refinement that the receiver's internal energy is affected by only minimum physical contact—for example, a hand placed lightly on the abdomen—or, in some cases, no actual contact at all. Traditional Chinese Medicine views the living body as a manifestation of universal energy. The physical form of the body is said to be surrounded by an invisible energy layer—a kind of "interface" between the material body and the entire energy of the universe. Therefore, it may be that those who are sufficiently attuned can, in some way, channel healing energy by gaining access to this layer.

Project energy

While this level of shiatsu practice may be beyond the scope of most, you will do no harm if you experiment with your ability to sense and project energy in this way. Hold your palm a few inches away from the area of the receiver's body you want to affect, and focus on sensing any lack or excess of energy. You could then try projecting your own healing energy as appropriate. Even if you do not achieve great results, you will have gained a deeper insight into the possibilities of shiatsu and perhaps an enhanced appreciation of the complexity and subtlety of the therapy you are using.

Universal Energy

According to ancient Chinese philosophy, physical matter in the universe is composed of energy. This philosophy is explained in detail on pages 10–33.

BASIC SHIATSU ROUTINE

Shiatsu does not lay down a fixed order of working: everyone develops their own program, according to personal preference and the needs of the person they are treating. The sequence suggested in this chapter includes only techniques that can be undertaken safely by a newcomer to shiatsu. It starts in the prone position, then illustrates a supine sequence, followed by a sequence for working on the side of the body. The final part of the chapter describes work in the sitting position. The whole routine need not be completed in one session, since this would be long and tiring for both parties.

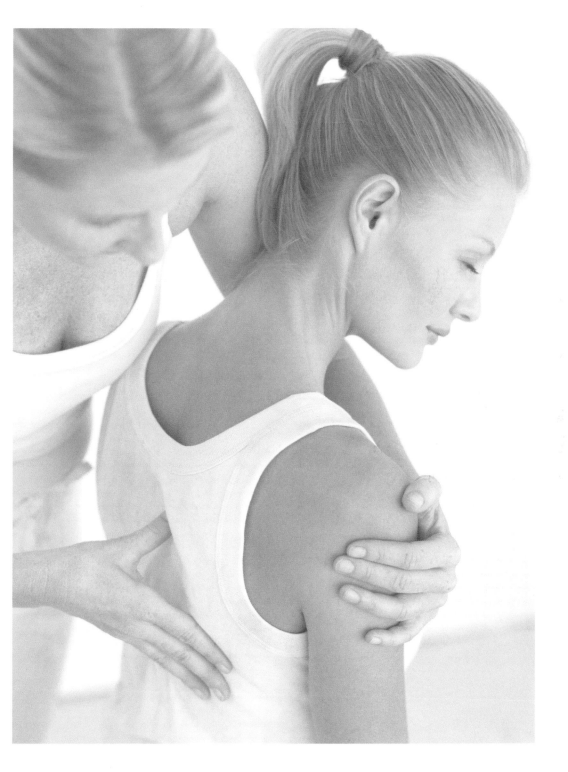

Prone Position

The prone position (lying on the stomach) is a good starting point for your shiatsu program. This position feels unthreatening and secure to most people. It is a natural tendency to protect your vulnerable abdominal organs by curling in and turning your back to defend yourself. It is a good policy to work with such basic instincts rather than adopting a more confrontational approach.

Back channels

The prone position allows access to the channels that run down the back of the body. The principal channel affected is the Bladder channel, which has two pairs of branches running down each side of the spine. It has a powerful integrating effect on all the organs, carrying downward yang energy from head to toe. The muscles of the back and shoulders are also commonly affected by stress and tension, so starting your routine using moderately strong pressure on this area has the advantage of relaxing the receiver, who will then be more receptive to the treatment that follows. Part of the Small Intestine channel is accessible at the shoulders and a section of the Kidney channel is also easily accessible as you work on the backs of the legs.

Receiver's position

Ask the receiver to lie on her stomach. Check that she is comfortable and place a pillow under the chest or abdomen,

Contact with receiver
Your first contact should be unhurried and reassuring.

if necessary. Turn her head to one side. Her arms should rest a little way from the sides of the body or may be placed under the head.

Giver's position

Sit in seiza next to her. Rub your hands briskly for about 30 seconds to encourage the flow of ki. Relax and rest your palm gently on her lower back and focus on sensing her breathing and energy flow. Remain in this position for a minute or so to accustom her to the contact. Your calmness and confidence will transmit to the receiver. Pay attention to your own energy center—your hara—and visualize how you are going to draw on this energy during treatment.

Cautions

Only work on those in good general health. Do not treat anyone who is pregnant, or who has a current acute illness, or a serious chronic condition. Do not work on any joint or tissue that is red, hot, swollen, or painful. Do not perform shiatsu if you are unwell yourself. Avoid giving or receiving shiatsu on a full stomach. If in doubt, do not treat.

STRETCHING THE SPINE

The first stage of back work involves applying simultaneous pressure to the upper and lower spine. This eases tense muscles and opens the Bladder channel. Pressure is conveyed equally through both hands, as they gently stretch the spine and flatten the lumbar curve. Use the knees-wide kneeling position to allow you to move your hara forward to apply the necessary pressure. Keep your back straight and your chest and shoulders open.

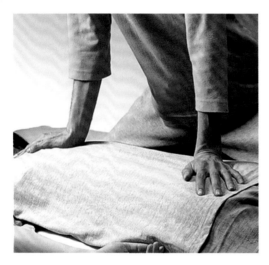

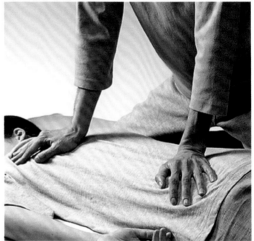

1 *Start the session with your hands on the top and the base of the spine. Lean forward to exert gentle pressure. Listen to the receiver's breathing and try to sense her energy flow. This gives a gentle stretch to the spine.*

2 *Use your weight to increase the pressure through both hands. Be aware of how the receiver responds. Move your hands, one at a time, to positions on the far side of the receiver's back, just below the shoulder blade and just above the buttock. Reapply weight to increase the pressure through both hands. Repeat on near side.*

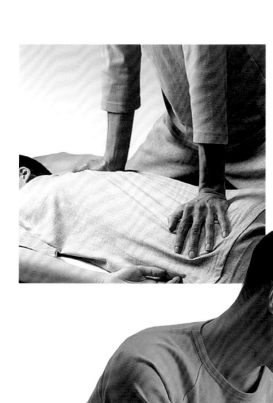

3 *Move your upper hand to the buttock farthest from you and the lower hand to the near shoulder. Lean over and exert steady pressure to stretch the back diagonally.*

4 *Reposition your hands so that they are crossed over the lumbar region—the lower hand on the sacral area and the other above the waist, under the ribs. Direct your weight to apply pressure that flattens and stretches the waist area.*

Body weight applies pressure

Hands crossed over lumbar region

Working the Bladder Channel

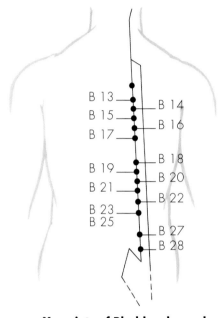

B 13
B 15
B 17
B 14
B 16
B 19
B 21
B 23
B 25
B 18
B 20
B 22
B 27
B 28

Yu points of Bladder channel
*The tsubos on the inner branch of the
channel can be manipulated to affect
energy flow to the different organs.*

The Bladder channel is now open and ready to receive more focused work. Keep in mind the twin pathways of the channel as you work on one side of the spine at a time. The inner branch closest to the spine has 12 tsubos, sometimes known as yu points, that represent sites at which Bladder energy feeds into the different organs.

As you apply pressure progressively down the channel, you are regulating the flow of energy to each of the organs. This boosts the whole system and harmonizes Bladder energy throughout the body. Familiarize yourself with the location of each point and the organs they serve. Ask the receiver to tell you if a point feels tender or sensitive, since heightened sensation over any of these tsubos may indicate an imbalance in that organ. This knowledge will help you gear your shiatsu to the receiver's specific needs (see also pages 174–215).

Upper
The upper part of the back—known in shiatsu terminology as the Upper Heater region—contains tsubos for the Lung (B 13), Heart Protector (B 14), Heart (B 15), Governing Vessel (B 16), and Diaphragm (B 17). These organs are concerned with the circulation of blood and ki throughout the body. B 17 is a particularly powerful point for strengthening the flow of blood.

Middle

The middle section—Middle Heater region—contains the tsubos for the organs that are responsible for the digestion of food and the distribution of nutrients throughout the body. These are the Liver (B 18), Gallbladder (B 19), Spleen (B 20), Stomach (B 21), and Triple Heater (B 22).

Lower

The lower part of the back—known in shiatsu terminology as the Lower Heater region—contains the tsubos for the Kidneys (B 23), Large Intestine (B 25), Small Intestine (B 27), and Bladder (B 28). These organs are related to reproductive functions, storage, and elimination of wastes.

WORKING DOWN THE BACK

For this section of the shiatsu routine you will start from the same position at the side of your partner as that in which you finished the last. You will be working using different types of pressure and hand positions down each side of the spine. Do not apply pressure directly over the spine itself. The pressure you use should be firm but not too forceful.

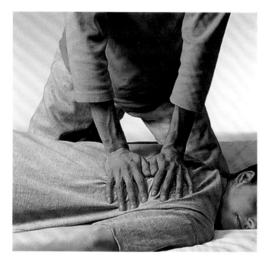

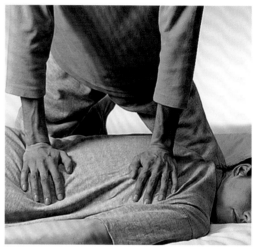

1 *Place one hand (the upper hand) between the spine and the shoulder blade farthest from you and the other hand (the lower hand) next to it.*

2 *Use the lower hand to palm down the back toward the sacrum, applying pressure through the heel of the hand. Make sure the upper hand remains passive.*

3 *Now repeat the previous two steps on the side of the spine nearest to you.*

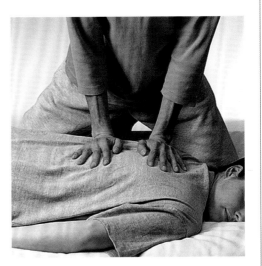

Underside of elbow
to buttocks

Supporting hand
on sacrum

4 *Use the flat underside of your elbow to apply careful, deep pressure around each of the buttocks in turn.*

The Lower Back & Shoulders

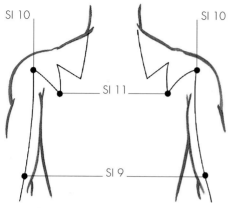

SI 10   SI 10

SI 11

SI 9

The Small Intestine channel

*Shiatsu treatment of this channel, which
zigzags over the shoulders, relieves pain
and stiffness in this area.*

Change position to work on the
lower back, adopting the lunge
position (see page 110). Here
you will be leaning into the sacrum—an
area that contains a large number of
tsubos on the Bladder channel.

Lower back

Pressure in this area can be very helpful
for those who are suffering from the effects
of poor posture and a sedentary lifestyle.
The lower back area is also a site for
strong emotions that in a modern, high-
stress environment are often pent up,
causing tension and frustration. Shiatsu
treatment of the lower back (according to
Traditional Chinese Medicine) can also
help alleviate problems arising from poor
circulation in the lower part of the body,
including varicose veins, menstrual
problems, and urinary tract disorders.

Shoulders

You are now ready to do some work
on the shoulders. Here you will be
manipulating the Small Intestine channel,
which zigzags across the shoulder blade
for part of its course. The Small Intestine
is concerned with separating the pure
from the impure: both food and fluids.
In this function it works closely with the
Spleen, Large Intestine, and Bladder.
There is also a psychological aspect to
the function of the Small Intestine, relating
to the ability to analyze and assimilate
information and sort the useful from the
unimportant. Work on this part of the
Small Intestine channel affects the head
and neck, and can have a strong local
effect, relieving pain and stiffness in the
neck and shoulders. It may also be useful
for those who are indecisive or whose
judgement is unsound.

At this stage in the routine you will
be using palm pressure. More intensive
treatment of these areas may be required
if a great deal of tension has accumulated
in the back and shoulders. You will return
to these areas to carry out more detailed
work with your thumbs later (see page
112). You have now treated the whole
back using different types of palm pressure.

(see page 112)

Caution

Take care when treating a painful neck or back
condition. If the receiver is suffering from pain in
the neck or back with pain, numbness, or tingling
in any limb, consult a doctor.

LOWER BACK & SHOULDERS
You are already well positioned for further work on the lower back. Use the lunge position, in which you face forward in a half-kneeling stance, with your kneeling knee next to the receiver's buttocks and the foot of the raised leg near her shoulders. This allows you to work energetically along the length of the back, without strain or loss of stability. You can use fairly strong pressure during this part of the routine, but maintain a constant awareness of the receiver's response to the treatment. As you work on the shoulders, keep in mind the location of the Small Intestine channel, and use your palms sensitively to work on any tsubos you find.

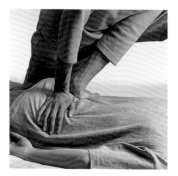 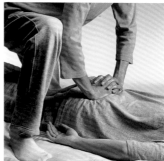 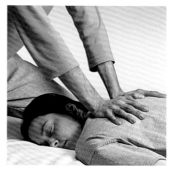

1 *In the lunge position, place both hands on either side of the spine at the waist. Shift your weight over your hands and "walk" your hands back toward the sacrum, bringing your hara back as you do so. Apply firm pressure to the sacrum.*

2 *Maintaining pressure on the sacrum for support, step astride the receiver. With your arms perpendicular to the sacrum, link your fingers and squeeze the heels of your hands together.*

3 *Keeping one hand on the receiver's back for continuity, move to her head, adopting a knees-wide position. Place both hands in the center of the shoulders and use your weight to exert firm palm pressure.*

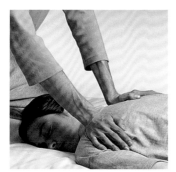

4 *Gradually move your hands away from each other, applying pressure along the shoulder and over the shoulder blades.*

5 *Kneel up and work with your palms down the sides of the back in parallel, moving your hara forward as you do so to maintain perpendicular pressure.*

Walk palms in parallel

Using Thumb Pressure on the Back

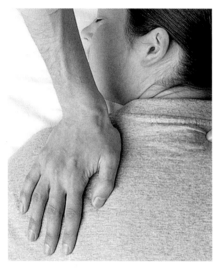

Precision work

Use of the thumbs on the back allows you to locate and treat the numerous tsubos that lie along the bladder channel.

Most people accumulate a great deal of tension in the back and shoulders and will appreciate a more intensive treatment. You may want to give special attention to particular yu points on the Bladder channel previously identified as being in need. Use your thumbs to work on Bladder and Small Intestine channels in the back and shoulder areas.

Shoulders

Begin this segment of the routine with the backs of the shoulders. You will not need to move from the position at the receiver's head in which you were working at the end of the last segment. Make sure you are comfortable and then rest both hands on the receiver's shoulders. Relax, breathe steadily and adjust yourself to the receiver's energy, before continuing.

You should familiarize yourself with the detailed course of the Small Intestine channel as it passes over the shoulder blade. There are several important tsubos in this area: notably Small Intestine 9, 10, 11, 12, 13, 14, and 15. Thumb these areas thoroughly if your partner complains of any pain experienced in the neck, the shoulder, or the arm.

Spine

The sequence then moves to areas on either side of the spine. The inner branch of the Bladder channel passes down the muscled ridge about one-and-a-half thumb-widths from the midline of the vertebrae. The yu points are on this branch of the Bladder channel. The outer branch lies about three thumb-widths from the midline. Position yourself so that your thumbs are angled at about 90 degrees to the back.

You will only be able to reach as far as the shoulder blades comfortably from your position at the head. Do not work further than this before changing position, to straddle the body, facing forward. Keep one hand in contact with your partner as you move into position. One of the skills of good shiatsu is to maintain your focus through these inevitable disruptions, when you have to pause to reposition yourself. This comes with practice both of shiatsu and related meditation techniques.

SHOULDERS & BACK
The position for this part of the routine is at the receiver's head. Kneel with your knees no farther forward than the receiver's ears. Use one hand to support one shoulder as you use the thumb of the other hand to work on the Small Intestine channel of the other shoulder. Then switch sides. When working the Bladder channel you will be using both thumbs together, working in parallel down the spine.

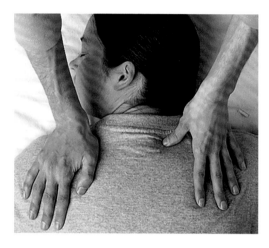

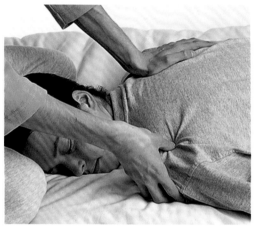

1 *Thumb along the path of the Small Intestine channel, down from the neck and across the shoulder blade. Use pressure sensitively to release any knots of tension you encounter.*

2 *The points on the outer shoulder, above the armpit, are particularly effective for countering neck and shoulder problems. Be sure to treat these thoroughly. Work on both shoulders.*

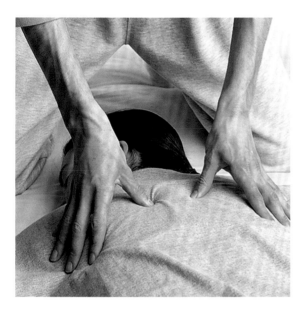

3 Use both thumbs in parallel to work the inner branch of the Bladder channel nearest the spine. Thumb from the neck to the middle back. Then work the outer Bladder channel along the crest of muscle on either side of the spine.

4 Kneel astride the receiver's lower back and thumb each branch of the Bladder channel from the middle to lower back. Then thumb the sacral area, in which many important Bladder tsubos are located.

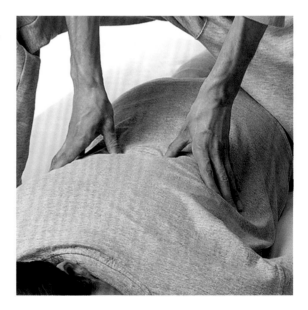

115

The Backs of the Legs

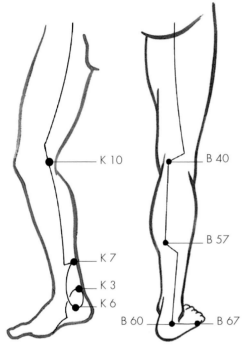

K 10

B 40

B 57

K 7

K 3

K 6

B 60

B 67

Bladder & Kidney channels

The Bladder channel carries yang energy down through the legs. The Kidney channel carries yin energy upward.

You are now ready to start work on the lower parts of the Bladder and Kidney channels as they pass down the backs of the legs. Both channels are associated with the Water element and their functions are strongly interrelated. The significance of the Bladder channel

has already been discussed. The Kidney channel conducts yin energy upward through the body. Kidney energy, which underlies a sound constitution, can become depleted in those who have demanding jobs. Kidney deficiency may manifest as urinary or reproductive problems, backaches, and thinning hair. Work on the Kidney channels may help generate a feeling of stability in those with an unbalanced lifestyle. Women with menstrual problems may benefit from attention to the Kidney channel.

Thigh

This routine starts at the top of the thigh. Adopt a knees-wide kneeling position next to the receiver's legs, so that you can reach the buttocks with one hand and the feet with the other. Keep a supporting hand on the sacrum as you first palm and then thumb the Bladder channel of the near thigh. Then palm the Kidney channel on the inner aspect of the far thigh. Follow this by thumbing down the channel. The inner thigh may be sensitive, so proceed slowly. Maintain pressure for several seconds, breathing deeply. Use your hara energy to give more effect to your shiatsu.

Lower leg

Moving to the lower leg, palm and then thumb the Bladder channel as it passes from the center of the calf and toward the outside of the ankle. Pressure on Bladder 40 (a tsubo known as Supporting Middle) at the back of the knee may be of particular benefit to those with back problems.

This part of the routine also includes work on the ankles and feet, which contain several tsubos, including Bladder 60 (Kun Lun Mountain) and 67 (Reaching Yin). Allow enough time to pay these tsubos proper attention.

Caution

Do not apply pressure over any area of the leg which is inflamed, painful, swollen, or shows evidence of varicose veins. Putting too much pressure on varicose veins could result in a blood clot.

BACKS OF THE LEGS ROUTINE

In the previous part of the routine, you were kneeling astride the receiver. Keeping one hand in contact with the sacrum, move to the side of the receiver, next to the upper thigh. In a knees-wide position, you can now work down the thigh. As you work from the upper to the lower leg, be aware of the need to adapt the amount of pressure you use. The backs of the thighs contain large muscles and are relatively strong in most people, but the backs of the knees and calves can be sensitive. Moderate your technique accordingly. It is important that there is sufficient padding under the receiver's legs to prevent discomfort. In this segment, complete steps 1 to 5 on one side of the body and then repeat on the other side.

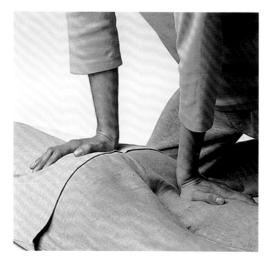

1 Rest one hand firmly on the sacrum. Place the heel of the other hand at the top of the center of the thigh nearest to you. Use your weight over your arm to apply pressure.

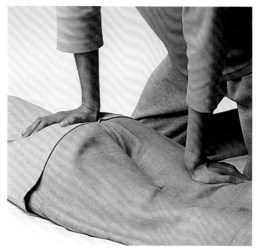

2 Move your active hand down the center of the thigh toward the knee in stages, applying firm pressure. Direct your energy from your hara, not your shoulder or back muscles.

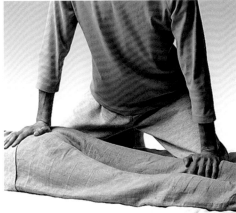

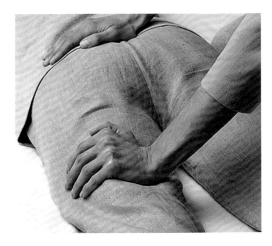

3 *Move your active hand to the top of the opposite leg. First palm down the inner aspect of the thigh and then use thumb pressure along the Kidney channel (this can be a sensitive area).*

4 *Palm down the back of the near leg. Follow the Bladder channel, remembering that it deviates from the center to the outer aspect below the calf muscle.*

Thumbing the
Bladder channel

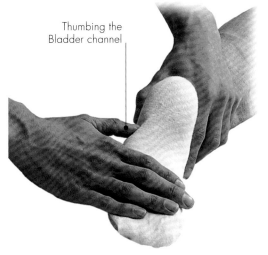

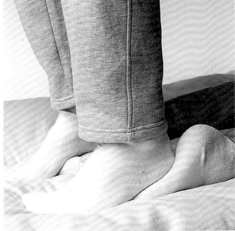

5 *Supporting the foot in one hand, thumb along the path of the Bladder channel on the outer edge of the foot. Now repeat the sequence on the other side.*

6 *Use your feet to apply pressure to the undersides of those of the receiver (for one technique, see page 95). Alternatively, apply increasing pressure with your heels.*

119

Leg Bending

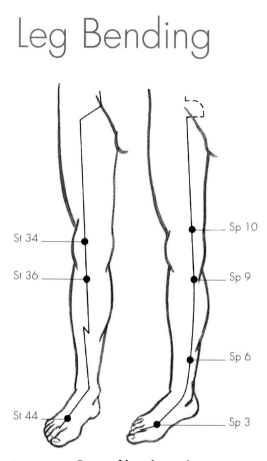

St 34

St 36

St 44

Sp 10

Sp 9

Sp 6

Sp 3

Front of leg channels
*Leg bending opens the Stomach channel
(left) and the Spleen channel (right),
improving energy flow.*

ntil now, the routine has relied on pressure techniques. Now we will turn to stretching and rotating, which are designed to improve mobility and to "open" the Stomach and Spleen channels in preparation for the work you will be doing later in the supine position. Both channels pass through the groin and are opened by exercises that stretch this area.

Stomach & Spleen

These organs are mainly concerned with nurturing and nourishment. Energy flow may be depleted in those whose life is centered around mental activities. Opening these channels improves the receiver's energy connection with the Earth, which lends an improved sense of grounding. The passive stretches described on the following page can also be helpful for those whose joints have become stiff, perhaps through a sedentary lifestyle. People who do not have the energy or strength to do stretching movements on their own may appreciate this form of bodywork.

Acceptable limits

Shiatsu stretches can feel both relaxing and energizing for the receiver, but you need to be sensitive to signals that indicate when you have reached the limits of the acceptable and safe range of movement. There are no easy guidelines: every individual has a different degree of flexibility in each of their joints. You need to work slowly without sudden increases in pressure that could result in injury for your partner. Never try to force a movement and always be prepared to stop the moment your partner indicates by word, facial expression, or other body signal that the stretch has reached its comfortable limit.

Manipulating heavy limbs can be tiring for you. Keep your weight "underside" as you lift and exert steady pressure. This lets you use minimum force to maximum effect. Work from your hara and use this energy rather than the muscle action of the arms to produce a cooperative response from your partner's body.

Caution

Take care when flexing the leg of any person who has a history of knee joint problems. Fully flexing the knee may cause pain or damage for people with such a history.

LEG BENDING ROUTINE

Working from the receiver's side as for the previous sequence, lift and maneuver the leg on the side you are working with one hand. Keep your passive hand resting on the sacrum throughout the sequence shown on this page. This gives stability by preventing the hips from shifting as you rotate the legs. It also provides an energetic connection that enhances the flow of ki.

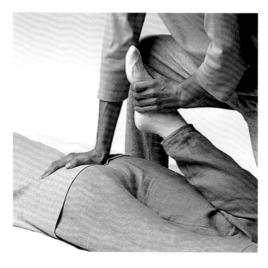

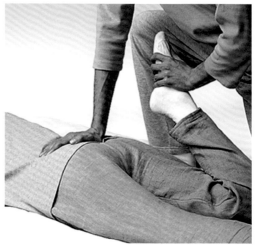

1 *Grasp the instep of the foot on the near side and bring it up over the buttock on the same side. Gently but firmly press the foot as close to the buttock as is comfortable.*

2 *Bring the foot back above the knee, then gently push it forward toward the outside of the buttock nearest to you. Do not take the stretch further than is comfortable.*

3 *Once again, bring the foot back. Now bring it toward the opposite buttock, pressing gently to achieve the maximum comfortable stretch.*

4 *Release the pressure to bring the foot back above the knee between stretches.*

Passive hand maintains contact

Supine Position

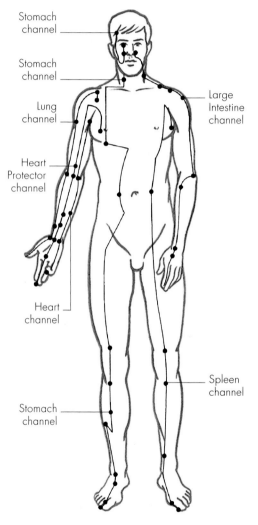

Stomach channel

Stomach channel

Lung channel

Heart Protector channel

Large Intestine channel

Heart channel

Stomach channel

Spleen channel

Front channels

The supine position allows access to the channels of the Lung, Large Intestine, Spleen, Stomach, Heart, and Heart Protector.

After you have completed the prone sequence, allow yourself and the receiver a moment or so before she moves into the supine position, lying on her back. Some of the main physical centers of emotion, such as the chest and abdomen, are now exposed, so your partner may feel more vulnerable. Make sure she is quite comfortable and be considerate in the way you position yourself. Sitting in seiza and facing forward at the receiver's side, relax your arm and place your hand over the receiver's navel. Spend a few moments sitting in hara and attuning yourself to the rhythm of the receiver's breathing before starting any specific treatments.

Lung & Large Intestine

The first stage of the supine sequence involves work on the arms, which contain the Lung and Large Intestine channels and parts of the Heart and Heart Protector channels. Both Lung and Large Intestine are concerned with vitality and the ability to transcend boundaries between the "self" and the "outside." The Lungs receive ki from the outside and distribute it around the body. Weakness of the Lungs leads to fatigue, breathlessness, susceptibility to colds and chills, and respiratory complaints in general. The Large Intestine is involved in the processes of elimination. Poor energy flow in this channel is implicated in a variety of symptoms, such as diarrhea, constipation, colds, and sinusitis.

Heart

The Heart channel is located along the inner aspect of the arm. Work on this channel may be of particular benefit to those who suffer from circulatory problems and poor temperature control.

Heart Protector

The Heart Protector channel works closely with the Heart. Work on this channel calms the mind and relaxes chest tension. It is of great value at times of emotional stress and in feverish illnesses.

ARMS & SHOULDERS ROUTINE

Before commencing work on the arms and shoulders, help your partner to release any tension that may reduce the effectiveness of your treatment. Pick up and gently shake the arm on which you are about to work and encourage them to let go of any tension. Repeat this until their arm feels loose and floppy. You are now ready to work on the arm channels in turn. It takes training and experience to locate the channels precisely, but by repositioning the arm in stages, as described, you will facilitate access to the arm channels.

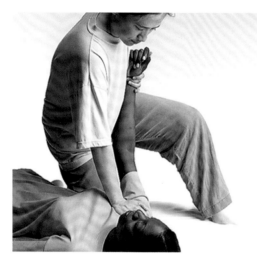

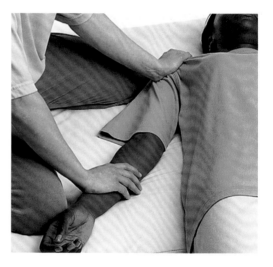

1 *Half-kneeling beside the receiver's shoulder, place your inside hand over her shoulder for support and pick up the arm with your other hand. Gently move it over your partner's head and then bring it around to the side. Take the arm only as far as is comfortable for your partner.*

2 *Place the arm at about 45° to her side, with the palm upward. Palm along the arm from the shoulder to the wrist. Then thumb along the Lung channel.*

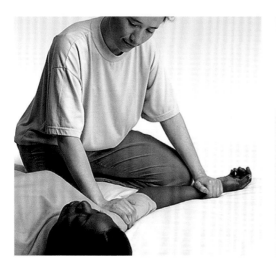

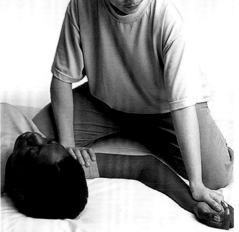

3 *Move the arm slightly further away from the receiver's side and palm, then thumb along the Heart Protector channel along the middle inside of the arm (see pages 124–5).*

4 *Move the arm comfortably above the receiver's head and palm down the Heart channel (see pages 124–5), which is accessible in this position.*

5 *Finish the routine by gently stretching and squeezing along the thumb and each finger from base to tip.*

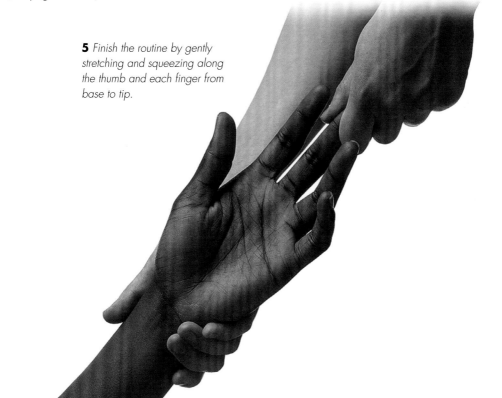

Face, Head & Neck

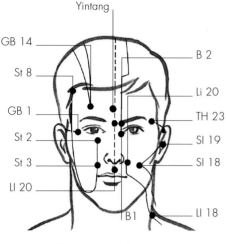

Yintang
GB 14
St 8
GB 1
St 2
St 3
LI 20

B 2
Li 20
TH 23
SI 19
SI 18
B 1
LI 18

Channels of the face

The face and neck contain a high concentration of channels and tsubos.

The supine position is ideal for working on the channels that pass through the face, head, and neck. The receiver can relax fully, without having to support the head in an upright position, and the giver can devote full attention to the application of suitable pressure, without needing constantly to adjust position. This routine is almost always welcomed by the receiver and can be used as a wonderfully soothing and energizing minishiatsu session on its own, if time is short.

Yang channels

Many channels are treated during this routine. These include sections of all the yang channels: Gallbladder, Small Intestine, Large Intestine, Triple Heater, Bladder, and Stomach. Some of the tsubos are of special importance for the sensory organs: B 1 (Eye Brightness) for eyes and vision; TH 21 (Ear Door) and SI 19 (Listening Palace) for ear problems; LI 20 (Welcome Fragrance) for nasal conditions.

Governing Vessel

The Governing Vessel is accessible through points on the head and face. This is one of the two channels (the other is the Conception Vessel) that run down the midline of the body. Unlike the other channels, which are paired on each side of the body, there is only one of each. The Governing Vessel extends from the base of the spine over the top of the head. It governs the yang channels and is linked to them all. Work on the Governing Vessel tsubos in the midline of the head and face has a powerful effect, lightening mood and improving clarity of thought. The tsubo on the Governing Vessel between the eyebrows, known as in-do, or Seal Hall, has a particularly harmonizing and calming effect.

Routine

When working on the face and head, in which many channels run close together, do not be overconcerned with identifying every tsubo accurately. You will probably gain access to them all if you work over the entire area following the natural, bony contours around the forehead and eyebrows, under the cheekbones, and along the jawline. Use your fingertips for most of this sequence: they provide the most suitable level of pressure with a reasonable degree of precision.

Shiatsu on the Head

Yang ki *may* accumulate in the upper body and head, leading to headaches, irritability, dryness, and flushed cheeks. Shiatsu on the head helps disperse excess yang ki effectively.

FACE, HEAD & NECK ROUTINE

Take up a position at your partner's head. Make sure that you provide a pillow to give support to the head and neck as you work. The first part of the routine relaxes the neck to allow the smooth flow of ki between the head and body. After you have done this, gently rest your hands on their temples to provide calm reassurance before starting work on the channels.

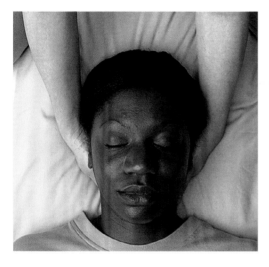

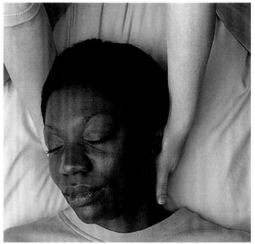

1 *Cradle your partner's head in your hands, with your fingers resting under the ridge at the base of the skull. Gently lift and pull to "open" the neck joints. This is a very subtle movement.*

2 *With your hands still resting under the head, slowly roll the head from one side to the other to loosen and mobilize the neck. Keep this movement gentle and smooth.*

3 *Resting the heels of both hands gently on the receiver's temple region, you can give relaxed fingertip pressure along the meridian lines and follow the contours of the face as shown. Work down the forehead, around the eyes and cheekbones, and into the corners of the nose. Emphasize any tsubos as you judge appropriate.*

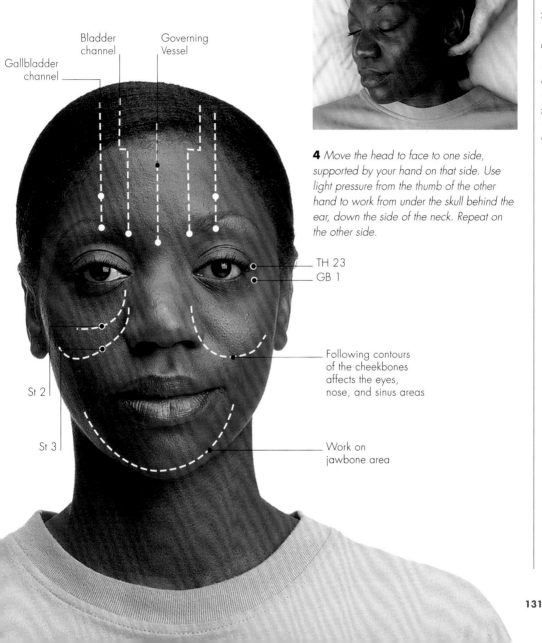

4 *Move the head to face to one side, supported by your hand on that side. Use light pressure from the thumb of the other hand to work from under the skull behind the ear, down the side of the neck. Repeat on the other side.*

Gallbladder channel

Bladder channel

Governing Vessel

TH 23
GB 1

St 2

St 3

Following contours of the cheekbones affects the eyes, nose, and sinus areas

Work on jawbone area

131

Hips & Legs

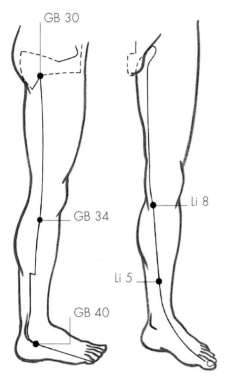

GB 30

GB 34

Li 8

Li 5

GB 40

Wood channels of the leg
*The Gallbladder channel (left) and
the Liver channel (right) can be treated
in the supine position.*

helps to promote strong connections with
the Earth, and cultivates nurturing.
Insecurity and irregular eating habits can
upset Earth energy, resulting in digestive
upsets and anxiety. Spleen disharmony
can also disrupt the menstrual cycle.

Routine & techniques

This segment also includes work on the
Gallbladder channel and the Liver
channel. Treatment of the Gallbladder
channel benefits those who cannot digest
fatty foods. Treatment of both of these
channels can provide generalized relief
for those who suffer from joint problems,
because the Wood element with which
they are associated governs the ligaments
and tendons. The techniques used include
stretches and rotations as well as palming
and thumbing. The legs are strong, and
you can use a fair degree of pressure.
However, take care when working the
Spleen and Liver channels in the inner
calf, because this area is often tender.
Check with the receiver and be prepared
to moderate your technique. Position
yourself carefully at each stage so that you
work from the hara, using a wide base.

Work on the hips and legs
focuses on the Earth channels
of the Stomach and Spleen.
These organs are concerned with the
digestion of food, so ki in these channels

Key Tsubos

While working on these areas you will encounter a number of important tsubos. The points relating to Stomach and Spleen are shown on page 120.

Sp 6, also known as Three Yin Meeting, is important for sexual function and menstrual disorders. Avoid in pregnancy.

Sp 10, also known as Sea of Blood, controls excessive bleeding.

St 34, also called Beam Mound, is useful for Stomach pains.

St 36, also known as Leg Three Miles, boosts the immune system and counters tiredness.

GB 30, also known as Jumping Circle, is useful for hip pain and sciatica.

GB 34, also known as Yang Mound Spring, relaxes stiff muscles and tendons.

Li 5, also known as Insect Ditch, is useful for emotional problems.

Caution

Be extra careful with any person who has a history of painful hip joints, or experiences any pain or discomfort when moving their hips. Do not use these exercises for any person who has had a hip joint replacement.

HIPS & LEGS ROUTINE

The first part of the routine focuses on mobilizing the hip joints. This opens the channels and helps to relax the hips and legs, making them more receptive to shiatsu pressure on the channels and tsubos. Using your elbow on the outer thigh is suitable and acceptable to most people, but if the receiver has a delicate physique or is elderly it may be prudent to substitute palm pressure.

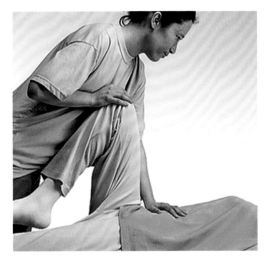

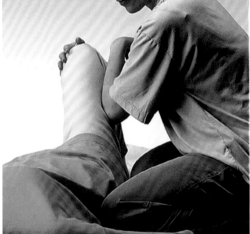

1 *Kneel next to the receiver's legs, facing her head. Place your outside hand on her hip for support. Raise the knee with your inside hand and gently rotate the hip joint in each direction. Encourage her to relax.*

2 *Support the receiver's bent knee in the raised position. With the flat underside of the elbow of the arm that was previously supporting the hip, apply pressure down the outside of the thigh.*

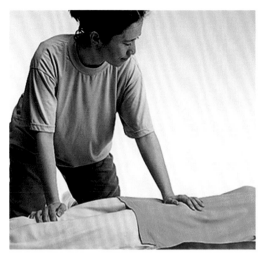

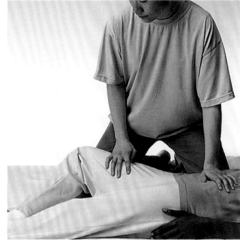

3 *With both legs stretched out, palm down the front of the leg, keeping one hand on the belly for support. Now position the receiver's leg so that her foot rests against her opposite ankle.*

4 *Rest the receiver's knee on yours for support. Keeping the passive hand on her belly, gently thumb down the inner aspect of the thigh and lower leg.*

5 *Reposition the receiver's leg so that the foot now rests against her knee. Place an extra pillow under the bent knee for support. With one hand on the opposite hip, press down on the bent knee to stretch the hip. Repeat steps 1 to 5 on the other side.*

Passive hand
stabilizes hip

The Feet

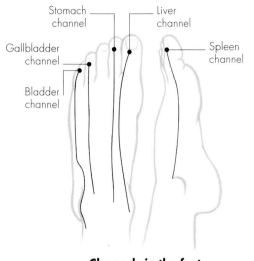

Stomach channel
Liver channel
Gallbladder channel
Spleen channel
Bladder channel

Channels in the feet

The presence of numerous channels and tsubos in the feet makes treatment of this area particularly powerful.

The feet carry our weight throughout the day, continually absorbing stress and acting as shock absorbers. They also provide the connection with the Earth's energy that we need for our sense of "wholeness." Shiatsu treatment of the feet provides an effective and welcome means of reviving tired feet, reopening channels that have become compressed through prolonged weight-bearing, and thereby enhancing the transmission of healing energy upward throughout the body.

The channels that either terminate or originate in the feet are the yang channels on the upper and outer surfaces—Bladder, Gallbladder, and Stomach—and the yin channels on the inner and lower surfaces—Kidney, Liver, and Spleen. Working the yang channels helps to draw down excess yang energy from the head and upper body, revitalizing and warming the feet. Working the yin channels opens them up to receive energetic stimulus from the Earth and encourages the upward flow of yin energy, which has a generally nourishing, calming, and cooling effect on the upper parts of the body.

Liver

The Liver channel in the foot, which starts inside the big toenail, has a special significance. A person who has been ingesting fatty foods and/or drugs (including medicines) and alcohol may suffer from Liver imbalance. This may lead to excess yang in the head, resulting in headaches and nausea. Excess Liver Fire, as this condition is termed, can be redressed by shiatsu pressure on the Liver channel in the foot.

Reducing sensitivity

This part of the body can be sensitive or even ticklish for some people. Start by thoroughly mobilizing the feet and ankles through gentle rotations, with the foot supported on your knee. When you handle the foot do it firmly, using the passive hand to provide reassuring support and connection.

Key Tsubos

Some of the key tsubos you will encounter as you work on the feet include:

Li 2, also known as Walk Between, is useful for headaches, menstrual pain, or urinary problems.

Li 3, also known as Great Pouring, is useful for increasing yin energy in the Liver, which nourishes tendons and ligaments and relieves stiffness.

K 1, also known as Bubbling Spring, is useful for calming yang and strengthening yin, which helps soothe an agitated state of mind.

St 44, also known as Inner Courtyard, is effective against stomach acidity and sore eyes or gums, as well as toothaches.

Sp 3, also known as Greater Whiteness, is useful for poor digestion, appetite loss, and diarrhea. This strengthens the neck and spine.

WORKING ON THE FEET

Take up a position at the receiver's side, level with the feet. Kneeling in seiza (see page 74) is the most effective stance. Work with the foot as close to your hara as possible. Provide a pillow for support under the leg on which you are working to keep the knee relaxed. The supine sequence ends with a heel-pulling exercise that stretches the spine, allowing the energy stimulated throughout the sequence to flow freely through the body.

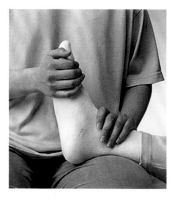

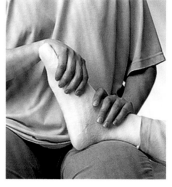

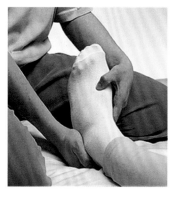

1 *Kneeling in seiza at the receiver's feet, rest his ankle on your knee. Stabilize the ankle with one hand, while you gently rotate the foot in each direction until you feel the ankle relax.*

2 *Exert firm pressure on the top of the foot, in order to stretch it downward. By holding the foot close to your hara, you are able to increase the effectiveness of the treatment.*

3 *Adjust your position to face the feet. Support the heel with one hand, and gently thumb the Liver, Stomach, and Gallbladder channels in the upper surface of the foot, down to the toes.*

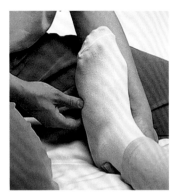

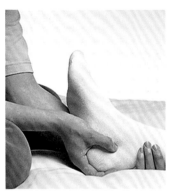

4 *Change hands to allow you to work more easily along the Bladder channel running down the outer edge of the foot.*

5 *Using one hand to support the ankle, thumb the Kidney and Spleen channels on the inner edge of the foot. Repeat steps 1 to 5 on the other foot.*

6 *When you have worked on both feet, stand at the receiver's feet, bend your knees to grasp both ankles from underneath, near the heels, and lift the receiver's feet, keeping your spine straight. Gently swing the legs from side to side. Then pull the ankles to stretch the spine. Keep your knees bent and hara low to avoid straining your back.*

Hara low

Knees bent

Side Position

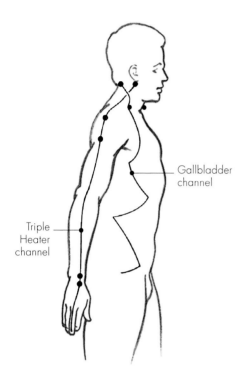

Side channels

*The principal channels accessed
from the side of the body are the Gallbladder
and Triple Heater.*

Gallbladder
channel

Triple
Heater
channel

The main part of the basic routine ends with the receiver lying on his or her side. This position allows you to gain access to the Triple Heater and Gallbladder channels. Sections of the Liver and Heart Protector channels, which have not previously been worked, are also reached easily.

Triple Heater

The Triple Heater channel distributes energy in three areas of the body known as the Upper, Middle, and Lower Heater regions, harmonizing the activities of the organs in those areas. Much of the activity of this "organ" is concerned with the processing and transportation of fluids. In the Upper Heater, fluids are transformed into vapor. Nourishing fluids are transported throughout the body from the Middle Heater. The Lower Heater processes and eliminates waste fluids. This concern with fluids provides a close link with the activities of the Kidneys. The Triple Heater also plays an important defensive role against environmental factors, such as cold and infection, leading to an association with the immune system. Shiatsu treatment of the Triple Heater channel gives an overall boost to the system, promoting the healthy flow of energy from the Kidneys throughout the body, providing a sense of warmth and well-being.

Gallbladder

The Gallbladder channel plays a key role in digestion and purposeful mental activity and works in close association with the Liver. Disturbance of these channels may lead to indigestion, joint and muscle stiffness, and frustration and indecision. Working on these channels enhances mental agility and creativity, as well as physiological functions.

Heart Protector

Working the Heart Protector channel benefits heart and circulatory function. It can also have tremendous mental and emotional effects, helping to overcome shyness or caution.

Before starting work, check that the receiver is comfortable, with the top leg bent and resting in front to provide stability. Use a pillow under the head and another under the knee and thigh of the bent leg. Choose a kneeling or half-kneeling position that enables you to complete the stretches without strain. Complete the entire routine (see pages 142–59) on one side of the body before asking the receiver to turn over.

SHOULDER & ARM ROTATION
The first stage mobilizes the shoulder joint to open the channels that pass through it and facilitates the free flow of energy between the arm and body. Stretching the arm both vertically and forward further relaxes and opens the shoulder area. Increase the stretches only gradually, working from your hara and looking out for indications of discomfort from the receiver. Your supporting hand is especially important because the shoulder is a complex joint.

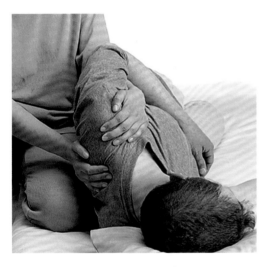

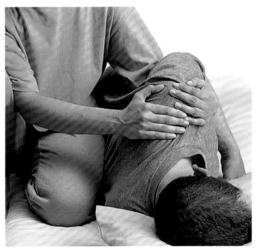

1 Support the front of the shoulder with the hand that is nearest the receiver. Place your other hand on his back, over the shoulder blade.

2 Hold the shoulder with both hands and rotate the shoulder a few times in each direction. Use the movement from your hara, not just your arms, to direct the rotation.

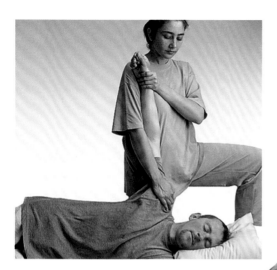

3 Keeping your nearside arm in contact with the receiver's shoulder, lift his arm up vertically. Grasp his wrist and pull upward slowly but firmly, without strain.

4 Bring the raised arm forward over the receiver's head. Adjust the position of the passive hand to stabilize the armpit, and pull the arm forward to stretch the shoulder.

Active hand provides pulling action

The Side of the Head

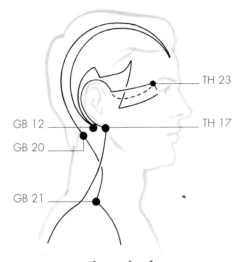

TH 23

GB 12

GB 20

TH 17

GB 21

**Channels of
the side of the head**
*The Gallbladder and Triple Heater
channels form complex pathways across
the side of the head.*

You have worked on the face and head in the supine position. In the side position, additional channels and tsubos are available for shiatsu treatment. These include points on the Triple Heater and Gallbladder yang channels along the side of the head and neck.

Some of these points occur where the bones in the skull join and can be felt as subtle indentations or areas of altered sensitivity. In addition to their effect on the energetic state of their channel, several of these tsubos have an important regulatory effect on sense organs or on localized problems affecting the neck and jaw.

Working the head

Work on the side of the head begins with palming the head, which opens the Triple Heater channel and the Gallbladder channel. When working on this area use gentle pressure that is evenly distributed across the palms. Give yourself enough time to attune yourself to the flow of energy through the channels before changing your position. With the channels open and receptive, you can now work with your thumbs along the base of the skull and along the convoluted path of the Gallbladder channel as it zigzags across the side of the head from the base of the skull to the brow and back again, and along the Triple Heater channel as it passes around the ear and across to the brow. While working, make sure that you support the back of the head with your passive hand. One reason why shiatsu on the head is so effective is that it helps harmonize any imbalances between yin and yang energies in the body. Yang ki collects in the upper body and head, causing unpleasant symptoms such as headaches, irritability, dryness of the mouth, nose, and throat, and flushed cheeks. Working on the head helps to disperse any excess yang ki.

Key Tsubos

Some of the key tsubos you will encounter in this sequence are:

GB 21, also known as Shoulder Well, for freeing tension in the head, neck, and shoulder. Avoid pressing this point during pregnancy.

GB 20, also known as Wind Pool, for all types of headaches, eye and ear problems, and nasal and sinus congestion.

GB 12, also known as Final Bone, for one-sided headaches and insomnia.

TH 17, also known as Wind Screen, for earaches, especially if caused by exposure to cold air.

SIDE OF THE HEAD ROUTINE

The side of the head incorporates several important blood vessels and nerves and gives access to the Triple Heater and Gallbladder channels. For this routine, apply only gentle pressure, using the flat of the thumb. Firmer pressure can be applied around the skull, provided this is acceptable to the receiver. Use your passive hand to provide support and connection at each stage.

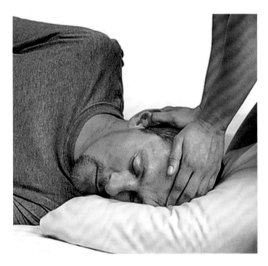

1 *With the receiver lying on his side, enclose the exposed front and side of the head with your hands. Remain in this position for a few moments, attuning yourself to the receiver's energy state.*

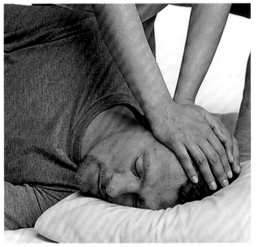

2 *Position yourself behind the receiver, facing his head. Keeping one hand at the back of the head, palm the forehead, temple, and upper jaw area with the other. Then gently thumb along the available channels on the side and back of the head (see page 144).*

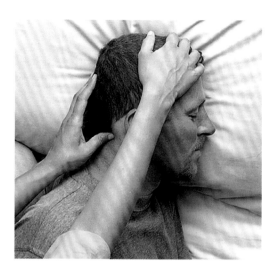

3 *Support the forehead with one hand, while you thumb along the channels behind the ear and along the base of the skull with the other hand.*

4 *Move the supporting hand to the shoulder and exert pressure to open the neck area. Use the flat of your thumb on the other hand to follow the Gallbladder channel down the side of the neck, behind the muscle that descends from the skull near the ear.*

Thumb follows Gallbladder channel in the neck

147

Outer Arm & Hands

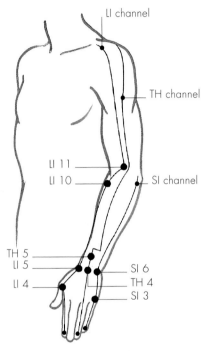

Outer arm channels
The Small Intestine, Triple Heater, and Large Intestine channels carry yang energy toward the head.

Labels on figure: LI channel, TH channel, SI channel, LI 11, LI 10, TH 5, LI 5, LI 4, SI 6, TH 4, SI 3

Withe the receiver still on their side, the next part of the sequence concentrates on the yang channels of the outer arm: the Small Intestine, the Large Intestine, and the Triple Heater. They are difficult, but general palming will influence them all

and more focused work on the hand will relieve many discomforts of the face, jaw, and sensory organs. The Triple Heater channel is the easiest to access, running down the middle of the outer arm, between the other two. Practice thumbing down this channel, which has significant positive local effects on the arm and shoulder, helping to relieve pain from strained muscles or ligaments.

Small Intestine
You will have already worked on the upper part of this channel as it traverses the shoulder blade. Treatment along the forearm may reduce anxiety or agitation.

Triple Heater
The important role of the Triple Heater channel in harmonizing the flow of energy between the upper and lower body is described on page 140. It is good to emphasize this channel if the receiver's Kidney ki is depleted. Working this part of the channel helps shoulder and arm pain. Further work may relieve headaches, earaches, eye irritation, and digestive or urinary troubles.

Key Tsubos

Important tsubos you will encounter include:

SI 3, also known as Back Stream, for strengthening the spine, relaxing muscles and tendons, and clearing the mind.

TH 5, also known as Outer Gate, for feverish conditions, sweating, and chills. Also for earaches, headaches, and swollen glands.

TH 4, also known as Yang Pond, for general boosting of ki. Also for pain in the wrist.

LI 11, also known as Crooked Pond, for cooling fevers and skin irritation.

LI 5, also known as Yang Stream, for wrist or thumb pain.

LI 4, also known as Meeting of the Valleys, for pain in the head, jaw, or teeth, strengthens yang ki generally, helping to fight off colds. It can promote contractions of the womb and should not be used in pregnancy.

OUTER ARM & HANDS ROUTINE

Your work on this part will involve palming, thumbing, stretching, and rotations. Check that the whole arm is relaxed before you start. Give it a gentle shake to release any tension. Rest the arm along the receiver's side as you work. Steady the shoulder with your passive hand. Use your thighs for additional support. The hands and fingers contain the terminal points for the channels you have been treating and several powerful tsubos.

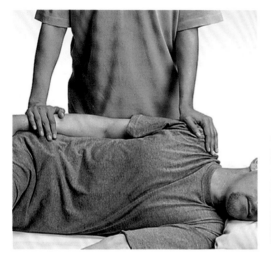

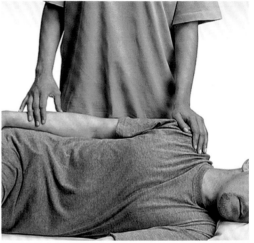

1 *Keep your passive hand in contact with the receiver's shoulder. Palm down the outer arm from shoulder to wrist, curving your hand to provide maximum contact.*

2 *Remaining in the same position, thumb down the Triple Heater channel from the shoulder to the fourth finger, then down the Large Intestine channel from the outer elbow crease to the forefinger (see page 148). Emphasize any tsubos that you encounter.*

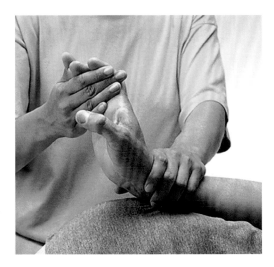

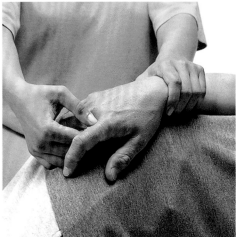

3 *Hold the arm just above the wrist and rotate the receiver's hand with your active hand. Do several turns in each direction to relax the joint and open the channels.*

4 *Maintain supporting contact with the passive hand. Now apply thumb pressure to the webs between the knuckle bones of the receiver's fingers.*

5 *Finish this part of the side routine by stretching each finger and thumb. Hold the wrist with one hand, and firmly grasp the base of the finger between your thumb and index finger. Work along the finger to the end.*

Finger squeezed
from base to tip

Passive hand
stabilizes wrist

Side Stretches

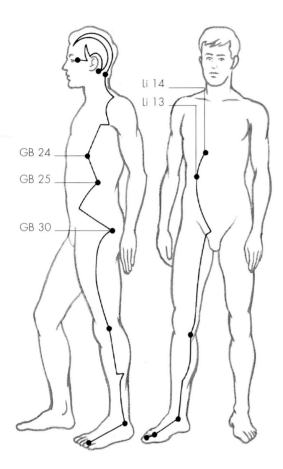

Li 14

Li 13

GB 24

GB 25

GB 30

The side channels
*Side stretches enhance the flow
of ki through the Gallbladder channel (left)
and the Liver channel (right).*

I n the side position you are able to gain access to the Gallbladder channel as it zigzags down the side of the torso, and to the short section of the Liver channel that surfaces at the side of the waist.

Gallbladder & Liver

Stretching the sides of the body opens both the Gallbladder and Liver channels and promotes the flow of ki in the chest and abdomen as a whole. It also contributes to the beneficial effects occasioned by having worked these channels in the feet (see page 136). The receiver should feel a pleasant sense of release in the waist, lower abdomen, and back.

All stretching movements, but particularly those of the sides of the body, promote the flow of Wood energy, which is the source of creative thinking and physical and mental flexibility. This is the element associated with growth and childhood, so there is a sense in which boosting this energy provides renewed vigor.

Positive pressure

Hand contact with the side of the body
can be ticklish for some people, but you
can minimize this by making any pressure
you apply positive and decisive. If you
convey a sense of uncertainty or if
your touch is tentative, the chances of
provoking a ticklish response in the
receiver are increased. Allow them to
adjust to your first contact before
continuing with treatment. Restrict yourself
to palming or Dragon's Mouth pressure,
a technique that uses the area between
the thumb and index finger (see page 81).
Encourage the receiver to breathe steadily
throughout the treatment. Try to keep your
hara aligned over the area on which you
are working. A raised or half-kneeling
position is preferable for this routine.

Dragon's Mouth

This technique is ideal for applying pressure to
curved areas such as the side of the body and
the arms, see page 81.

SIDE STRETCHES ROUTINE

Make sure the receiver is stable and comfortable in the side position, with the top leg in front of the lower one. Ask him to place his arms above his head or in front of him—whichever he prefers. The aim is to provide a relaxing and energizing stretch of the waist area, which is often restricted or compressed during normal activities. Allow enough time for you and the receiver to sense the ki flowing freely through the side channels. Some people find palming along their sides unbearably ticklish, so in such a case omit that part of the routine.

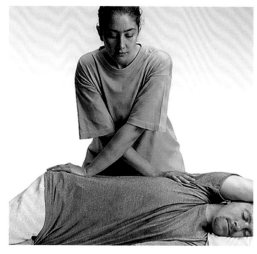

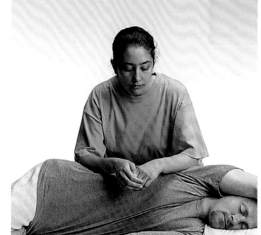

1 *Place yourself at the receiver's waist in an upright, knees-wide position. Cross your arms, placing one hand above the receiver's hip and the other above the waist. Lean from your hara to stretch out the waist.*

2 *An alternative to step 1 is to use pressure applied through the undersides of your forearms, which are placed above and below the waist. Maximize your effectiveness by using your hara energy as you lean in and roll your forearms apart. Try repeating in slightly varied positions.*

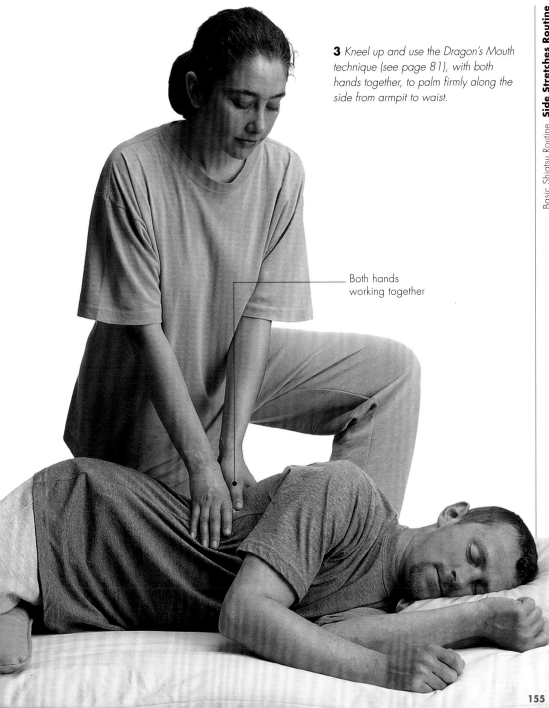

3 *Kneel up and use the Dragon's Mouth technique (see page 81), with both hands together, to palm firmly along the side from armpit to waist.*

Both hands
working together

Inner & Outer Leg Channels

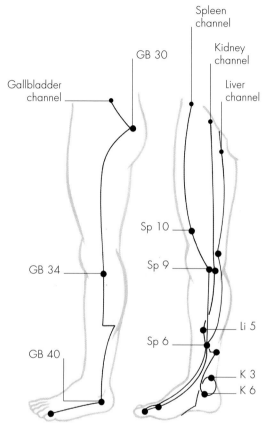

Spleen channel

Kidney channel

GB 30

Liver channel

Gallbladder channel

Sp 10

Sp 9

GB 34

Li 5

Sp 6

K 3

K 6

GB 40

Leg channels

Work on the yang Gallbladder channel (left) is balanced by treatment of the yin channels: Liver, Spleen, and Kidney (right). See also page 132.

The next stage of the routine continues in the side position and treats the channels of the inner and outer leg. The outer aspect of the leg contains the Gallbladder channel. This is the yang channel of the Wood element. Wood is associated with the health of the tendons and ligaments throughout the body.

The Gallbladder channel in the leg has several tsubos that have a particular relevance to the joints and general discomfort or stiffness in the muscles. Work on this channel may therefore be of benefit for people who participate in sports or who suffer from longstanding joint disorders such as arthritis.

Yin channels

Work on the Gallbladder channel is balanced by work on the yin channels of the inner leg. The Liver channel (the yin channel of the Wood element) runs between the Kidney and Spleen channels. It has wide-ranging functions largely concerned with the storage of blood, the nourishment of the muscles, and the regulation of the body's natural cycles, including menstruation. Work on this channel also contributes to the functioning of muscles and joints. The Kidney channel, toward the back of the inner leg, is of special importance for general constitutional strength and supports the work of all other organs.

The Spleen channel is nearest the front of the leg, and work on it improves the flow of Spleen energy, which has a toning role in the body. Weak muscles, a bloated abdomen, or a tendency to excessive bleeding may be helped by shiatsu treatment of this channel.

You have now completed a thorough shiatsu treatment. The next section describes work carried out in the sitting position (an alternative to lying down, more suitable for some people). If this does not apply to you, finish your session as advised on pages 172–73.

Caution in Pregnancy

The yin channels of the inner leg can have a powerful effect on the uterus. Do not work on these channels in anyone who is pregnant.

INNER & OUTER LEG ROUTINE

Bend the knee of the receiver's upper leg and rest it on a pillow in front of the lower leg so that his upper hip is angled forward a little. Check that he is comfortable and relaxed. When working on the hips and outside of the thigh, you can apply fairly strong pressure, using the elbow. If, however, the person you are treating has a delicate physique, be sure to moderate your technique: use lighter elbow pressure or use your palms instead. You will also be working on the inner leg. Remember that this area is sensitive for some people and adjust the pressure you use according to your partner's response.

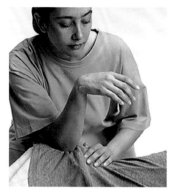 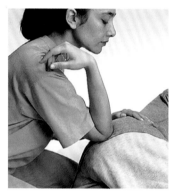 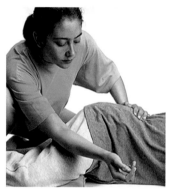

1 *Supporting hand on the hip, use the flat underside of your elbow to apply pressure into the buttock muscle, behind the hip bone. Listen to the receiver's response as you gradually increase pressure.*

2 *Vary your elbow pressure over the receiver's buttock area. Make sure that you lean in from your hara, and do not rely on force from your shoulder.*

3 *Use the underside of your elbow to apply pressure down the outside of the thigh. Position yourself as close to the area as possible to avoid strain.*

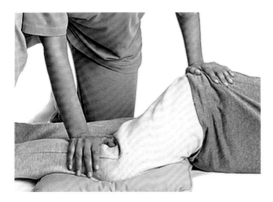

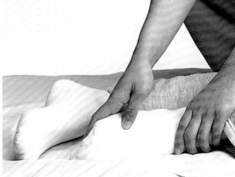

4 *Adjust your position, first palm and then thumb down the outer aspect of the lower leg, from the knee to the ankle. Pause at any tsubos you encounter.*

5 *Continue thumbing, moving onto the feet, and work the web between the fourth and fifth toes, the last points of the GB channel.*

6 *With your active hand turned outward, palm down the inside of the receiver's lower leg from he thigh to the ankle.*

Passive hand
provides support
at the hip

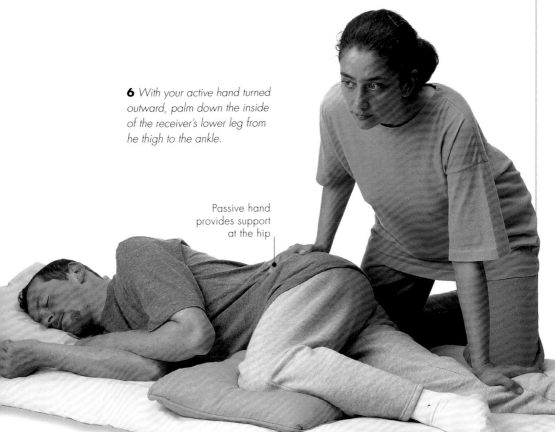

Sitting Position

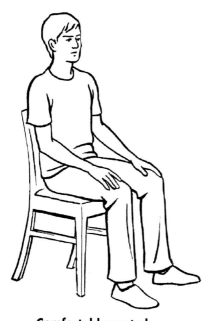

Comfortably seated

Work in the sitting position is suitable for shiatsu when floor work is not an option.

Different positions

Work in the sitting position includes sitting on the floor—kneeling or cross-legged—and sitting in an upright chair. A variety of different positions are illustrated on the following pages. The factors that you need to take into account as the giver of the treatment are: the suppleness and strength of the receiver, the areas of the body on which you intend to work, what positions you will need to use to apply pressure, and how you are going to give support to the receiver in your chosen position. Once you have mastered the basics, experiment with working in different positions. This will help you to develop your individual judgement and broaden the scope of your practice.

Reaching channels

In this section, you will learn how to give beneficial treatment to the neck, shoulders, and back with the receiver seated. But that does not mean that these are the only channels that can be given shiatsu from this position. You can easily gain access to the channels in the foot and lower leg with the receiver seated in a chair. All the channels in the hands and

Many people find it more comfortable to receive shiatsu when they are in a sitting position. Elderly people, for example, or those with joint problems or arthritis, may find it difficult to get down onto the floor and, perhaps more importantly, to get up again afterward. Asthma sufferers often find it easier to breathe deeply when in an upright position.

arms can be reached from any of the suggested sitting positions.

One of the great advantages of this therapy is that it is extremely adaptable. As you become more experienced, you will develop your own methods for treating different channels in different positions. Once you have learned to master the basics, experiment with working in different positions and this use of your individual judgement will broaden the scope of your practice.

Shiatsu at Work

If you are performing shiatsu at work and the floor is unsuitable, the sitting position provides a convenient alternative, allowing access to a surprisingly large number of channels.

OTHER SITTING POSITIONS
When selecting a suitable position, remember that shiatsu cannot be fully effective if the receiver is tense or uncomfortable. This will impede the free flow of ki. Use cushions to provide support, and be prepared to adapt your practice to the needs of the receiver. If you choose to work with the receiver in a kneeling or cross-legged position, they may need opportunities to get up and stretch if his or her legs become stiff or numb during treatment.

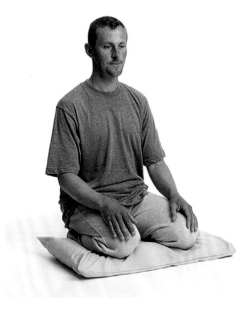

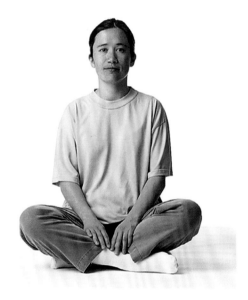

Kneeling
This position allows full access to the back and shoulders. However, some people find that it places a strain on the knees. A cushion can make the receiver more comfortable.

Cross-legged
Some people find this a relaxing position. It allows access to the back and shoulders and is quite stable. But for many people this is not a comfortable option.

Sitting on a stool

Sitting on a chair or stool is usually the preferred position for those with stiff joints. The giver of shiatsu needs to work in a standing position.

Astride a chair

If you are using a chair with a back, it may be necessary to have the receiver sit astride it, facing the chair back when you want to work on the shoulders and back. She can lean forward on the chair back for support.

163

Back & Shoulder Work in Sitting Positions

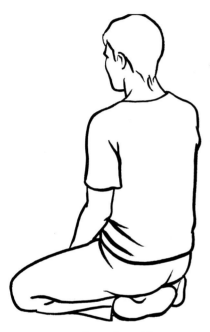

Preferred position

The most effective positions for this routine are kneeling or cross-legged. Provide a cushion for extra comfort.

This sequence provides welcome relief from pain and stiffness in the neck, back, and shoulders. It can be used as a "quick fix" in the office, or the treatment can be integrated as part of a longer routine. It allows powerful treatment of the yang channels that run across the shoulders: Gallbladder, Triple Heater, and Small Intestine. In addition, regulating yang ki can help to dispel symptoms such as headaches and congestive conditions of the head area. Avoid strong downward pressure on the shoulders in anyone who is pregnant as it may provoke miscarriage.

Techniques

You will mainly be using blunt pressure with the palms and elbows to ease tension by gently stretching the large muscles of the back and shoulders. You can also thumb the various channels if you want to provide a more intensive treatment of these areas. GB 21 in the center of the top of the shoulders is an important point for improving the downward flow of yang ki and releasing stiff neck and shoulders. Do not press this point during pregnancy. Keep thumb pressure at right angles to the area worked. The sequence also includes a relaxing neck stretch, which must be performed with great care. The neck stretch is achieved by the weight of the receiver's head acting on relaxed muscles. There should never be any pressure from the giver, which could cause injury to the vulnerable structures of the neck.

Position

The best position for back and shoulder work is one in which the receiver is either kneeling or cross-legged on the floor; this allows you to apply strong downward pressure on the shoulders in a half-kneeling stance, while using your thigh to support the receiver's back. Start by sitting behind the receiver. Place your supporting hand on one shoulder and slowly work down the spine, using gentle pressure from the palm of your active hand. This will provide a reassuring first contact and help you gain a sense of the receiver's overall condition.

BACK & SHOULDER ROUTINE

The best position is one in which the receiver is either kneeling or cross-legged on the floor—this allows you to apply strong downward pressure on the shoulders in a half-kneeling stance, while using your thigh to support the receiver's back. Start by sitting behind the receiver. Place your support hand on one shoulder and slowly work down the spine, using gentle pressure from the palm of your active hand. This will provide a reassuring first contact and help you gain a sense of the receiver's overall condition.

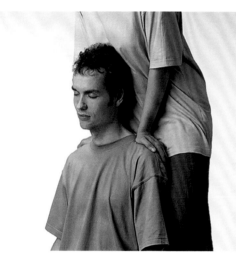

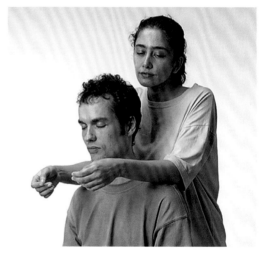

1 *From a standing position, place your palms on the receiver's shoulders. Exert steady downward pressure from the neck outward. Do not perform this step if the receiver is pregnant.*

2 *An alternative to palm pressure is to use the underside of your elbows. In a raised half-kneeling position, as close to the receiver as possible, place your forearms on his shoulders. Relax your arms and lean into the shoulders.*

3 *Support each shoulder in turn with your outer hand and apply pressure with your elbow along the back of the shoulder, working outward from the base of the neck.*

4 *Support his forehead with one hand. Now lift the head a little and remove the supporting hand, allowing the head to drop forward; catch it with the other hand. Repeat a few times.*

5 *Encourage the receiver to allow the neck to relax and drop forward. Continue to support the forehead with one hand. Place the other hand on the neck and gently move the head from one side to the other.*

Neck relaxed

Neck & Back Stretches in Sitting Position

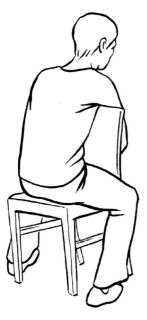

Chair support
A chair back provides good support for back work carried out in a sitting position.

The shiatsu sequence illustrated on the following pages is a sitting version of the back treatments carried out in the prone position. It provides a thorough treatment of the Bladder channels on each side of the spine using both palming and thumbing techniques. See also page 104 for further detail.

Spine stretch

The first element is a satisfying stretch of the spine, using diagonal pressure on the buttock and opposite lumbar area. This requires the receiver to adopt a kneeling pose. If the receiver finds this difficult, then omit this stage. You will need to judge how much pressure to exert and choose your technique accordingly. If the receiver is strong, straddle the back and use the pressure of your weight transmitted through your hands to stretch the spine. If you judge that this position may be too forceful for the receiver, choose a gentler stretch using your forearms.

Working the spine

For the next stage of the treatment the receiver can kneel, sit cross-legged, or sit on a chair. In the first two cases, work with one hand and hold the other hand across the front of their chest and shoulders for support. Use the thumb and knuckle of your index finger to exert simultaneous pressure on both sides of the spine. This helps open the chest and promote good breathing, as well as benefiting the back.

If the receiver is sitting on a chair, ask him to turn around and sit astride facing the back of the chair. He can then use the chair back for support, freeing your hands to work together down the spine.

Shoulders

In the closing stages of this sequence, return to treatment of the shoulders.

Squeeze the muscles from the base of the neck to the tips of the shoulders several times until they feel relaxed and free from tension. Then extend this squeezing action down the upper arms. Complete the sequence with a soothing, stroking action from the shoulders to the elbows to harmonize the flow of ki.

NECK & BACK STRETCHES Step 1 of this sequence requires

the receiver to adopt a kneeling position. If he finds this uncomfortable, omit this stage. You will need to judge how much pressure to exert and choose your technique accordingly. If the receiver is strong, straddle the back and use the pressure of your weight, transmitted through your hands, to stretch the spine. If you judge that this may be too forceful for the receiver—either because you are relatively heavy or he or she is of delicate build—choose a gentler stretch using your forearms. The remainder of the steps can be done with the receiver either kneeling or sitting in a chair.

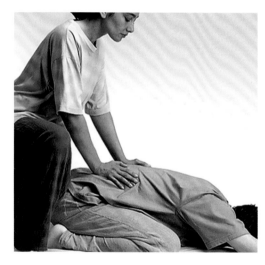

1 *Stand astride the receiver and place one hand above his hip on one side, and the other above the waist on the other side. Apply pressure (see above). Repeat with hand positions reversed.*

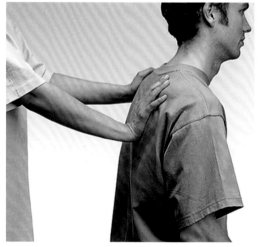

2 *With the receiver in an upright seated position, support one shoulder with one hand and palm down the back on the same side with the other. Repeat with hand positions reversed on the other side.*

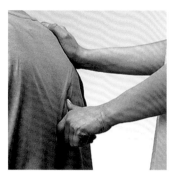 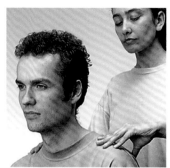

3 *Place one hand on the receiver's shoulder for support, then thumb down the Bladder channel on that side next to the spine from shoulder to waist (follow pathway as shown for back routine on pages 114–15). Repeat on other side, changing hands.*

4 *Thumb along the back of the shoulder (see pages 114–15). Then use both hands to squeeze along the length of both shoulders simultaneously from the neck outward.*

Brushing down the upper arms

5 *Finish the sequence by brushing down the upper arms from the shoulder to the elbow several times. Then pause with your hands resting on the receiver's back.*

After the Session

It is important to complete your shiatsu session with the same care and sensitivity with which you started. This enables the receiver to assimilate the effects of the treatment and the giver to break contact gently but completely.

Ending the session

In most cases, the best way to finish is as you began—sitting in hara for a few moments, focusing on the flow of ki within the receiver's body. You may prefer to sit at the receiver's head with your hands resting on his forehead. In either case, after a few moments smoothly remove your hands and cover the receiver in a light blanket so that he can continue to relax for a couple of minutes. After this time advise him to get up slowly. This is important because many people feel a little lightheaded or unsteady on their feet after a shiatsu session, and some practitioners advise people to avoid driving immediately afterward. If necessary, allow the receiver to remain sitting for a few minutes longer until he feels he is mentally and physically ready to resume everyday activities.

Separation techniques

It is equally important for the giver of shiatsu to end the session properly since shiatsu can be physically and mentally draining. After the session, separate yourself from that contact and then recharge your own energy. Restore your own ki by taking some deep breaths and/or performing some makko-ho stretches for the Lungs. A popular separation technique is to wash your hands after a session. This is sensible if you are a professional, treating several

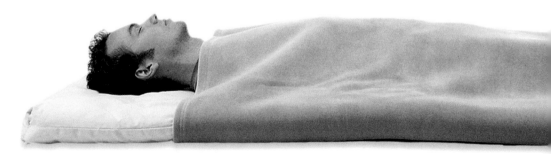

patients in succession, although the risk of transmitting any infection is minimal.

Aftereffects

If you plan to give further shiatsu treatments, ask the receiver to make a note of how he feels both physically and mentally in the days following the treatment. This will help you gauge the efficacy of your treatment and to plan subsequent ones. Also remind him of shiatsu techniques he can use at home, such as makko-ho and self-treatment of specific tsubos.

Relaxation time
After the shiatsu session, it is important to let the receiver relax for a few minutes before getting up.

SHIATSU
FOR HEALING

Shiatsu works best when used regularly as an integral part of a healthy lifestyle but it also provides an effective treatment option for a wide variety of disorders and symptoms. This chapter contains instructions on how to treat the relevant tsubos and channels in order to redress the possible imbalances that may lie at the root of the problem. Many of the treatments can be self-administered, although you may occasionally need someone to help you because it is not possible to reach all the points. Get a medical diagnosis for any symptoms for which you would normally seek your doctor's advice and in all cases of persistent, unexplained symptoms. Inform your doctor that you are using shiatsu in conjunction with orthodox treatments.

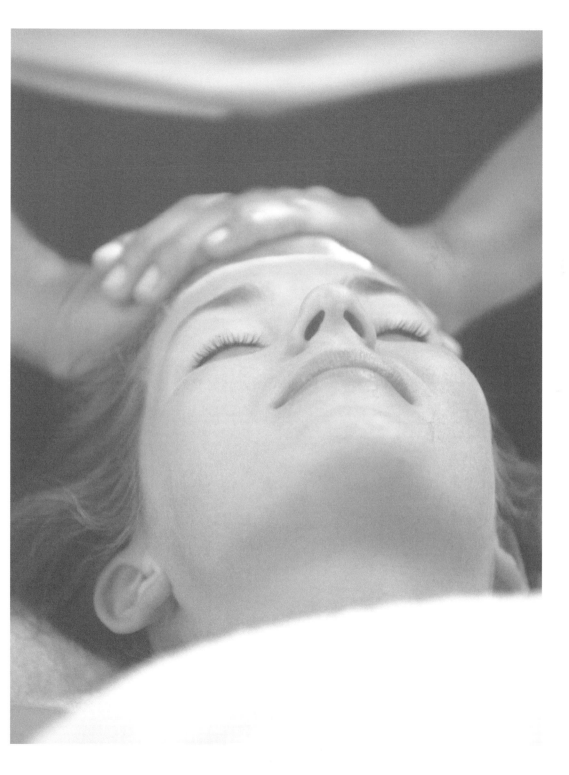

Respiratory Disorders

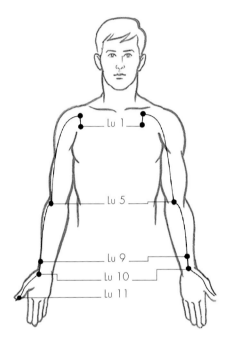

The Lung channel
Work on the Lung channel is helpful for all respiratory disorders. Work this channel on both sides of the body.

Respiration includes the process of drawing air into the lungs, so that oxygen can be absorbed into the bloodstream, and the complementary process of expelling waste gases from the body. In TCM air provides one of the three forms of ki. The Lungs govern the intake of air ki and are our first line of defense against climatic influences and other threats. Lung weakness can lead to frequent colds, coughs, and other forms of breathing problems. For all respiratory problems try to strengthen Lung ki by working on the Lung channel in the arms and hands. Do this carefully, emphasizing any tsubos you encounter along the channel. Practice the makko-ho stretch for the Lung channel every morning. Treating the generally energizing point CV 6 and the immune system booster St 36 can also be effective for all respiratory problems.

Upper respiratory tract

For symptoms affecting the upper part of the respiratory tract, such as colds, sore throat, and sinus congestion, treat the channels in the head and face, working under the eyes and along the cheekbones. Working the Large Intestine channel can also help. LI 4, Great Eliminator, is a particularly important point for strengthening your defenses and alleviating a runny nose, sneezing, and streaming eyes (NEVER use this point in pregnancy). There are two special points that are helpful for sore throats. Lu 10 (also known as Fish Border) at the base of the thumb and Lu 11 at the tip of the thumb should be given special emphasis as you work the Lung channel as a whole.

Lower respiratory tract

Coughs, wheezing, and other symptoms related to the lower respiratory tract, the windpipe, and lungs benefit from treatment of the yu points on the Bladder channel in the upper back. Working on CV 17 in the center of the chest, either by tapping the chest with your fist or by pressing on the point, may help to release tightness in the chest (and pent-up emotions). For asthmatics, treat the paired *ding chuan* points called Stops Wheezing.

Caution in Pregnancy

Large Intestine 4, Great Eliminator, exerts a powerful downward action and must not be used if the receiver is pregnant.

TREATMENT ROUTINE

The Lungs are particularly vulnerable to dryness and are also weakened by the effects of pollution and a poor diet. Choose the channels and tsubos you will treat according to the symptoms you are experiencing. You will need a helper to treat the Bladder channel in the upper back. Work on these areas once or twice a day, or more frequently if you find it helpful. Seek immediate medical attention if you experience severe breathlessness.

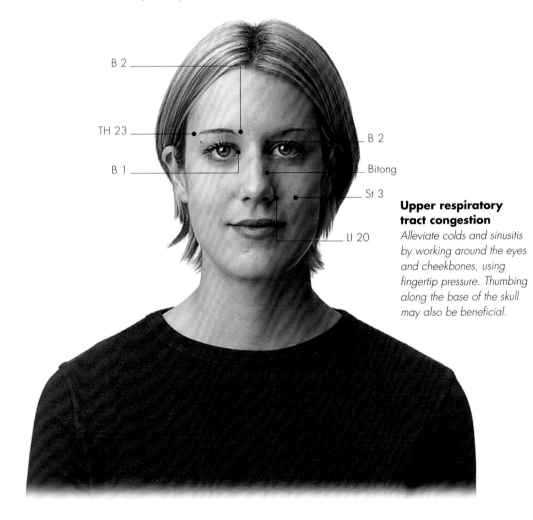

B 2

TH 23

B 1

B 2

Bitong

St 3

LI 20

Upper respiratory tract congestion

Alleviate colds and sinusitis by working around the eyes and cheekbones, using fingertip pressure. Thumbing along the base of the skull may also be beneficial.

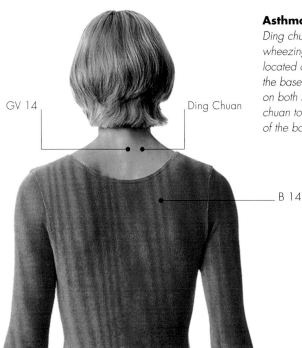

GV 14

Ding Chuan

B 14

Asthma & wheezing

Ding chuan is a special point for wheezing conditions. There are two located on each side of the spine at the base of the neck. Thumb in parallel on both sides of the spine from ding chuan to B 14. GV 14 in the midline of the back is also useful for coughs.

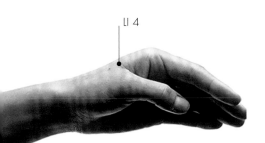

LI 4

Expelling wind & damp

Many upper respiratory conditions, particularly those with sneezing and streaming eyes and nose, respond to treatment of LI 4. Never use this point in pregnancy.

Sore throat

Work on Lu 10 and 11 in the hand is recommended for this symptom.

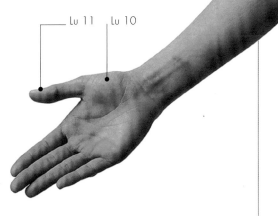

Lu 11   Lu 10

Indigestion & Nausea

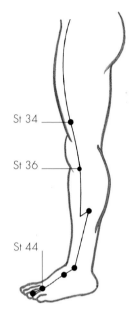

The Stomach channel

Work on this channel is helpful for most upper digestive tract problems.

St 34

St 36

St 44

Disharmony in the Stomach channel may cause its normal downward flow of energy to reverse and flow upward, resulting in nausea and vomiting. Stomach disharmony also has a psychological aspect. Anxiety and excessive mental stimulation without sufficient care for the body's physical needs are often associated with indigestion and feelings of nausea.

For all upper digestive problems, treat tsubos on the Stomach channel away from the abdomen, which may be too tender to tolerate pressure. Points on the leg are often the most useful. Work on the Spleen and Gallbladder channels at the same time.

Pain

If you are suffering from acute pain, apply thumb pressure to St 34 (Beam Mound), found just above the outside of the knee. For heartburn, acid indigestion, nausea, and vomiting, work on St 44 (Inner Courtyard). This tsubo is also useful for gum problems and toothaches. In addition, treat St 36 (Leg Three Miles). This point generally strengthens the digestive system and in particular helps

E astern and Western medical theory agree that an upset stomach leading to pain in the upper abdomen and/or nausea and vomiting is often caused by overindulgence in rich food. In shiatsu the problem is usually addressed by working on the Stomach and Spleen channels (both organs of the Earth element) and in some cases the Gallbladder channel (Wood element).

the Stomach and Spleen transform food into blood and ki, thereby relieving stagnation in the Stomach.

Nausea

HP 6 (Inner Gate), found on the inside of the wrist, is an important and highly effective point for treating nausea of all kinds, including motion sickness. This tsubo has a calming influence on the chest and abdomen and helps to harmonize the Stomach.

For upper abdominal pain that is not accompanied by nausea or vomiting, try using gentle finger pressure under the ribs, working outward from the center. Circular massage of the abdomen may also be soothing.

If someone is available to help, ask them to work on the yu points governing the digestive system on the Bladder channel in the middle of the back. Emphasize B 17 to B 21 on both sides of the spine.

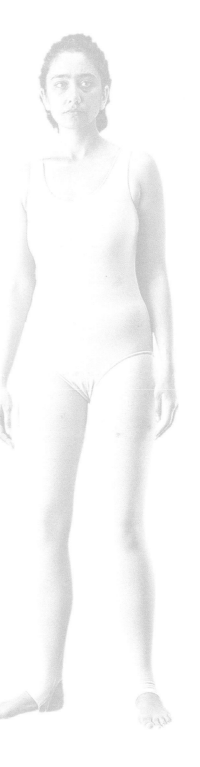

TREATMENT ROUTINE

Try working the channels and tsubos described here if indigestion and/or nausea are common problems for you. You may find it more acceptable or effective to work some of these areas when symptoms have abated. This will help to strengthen your system and prevent a recurrence of the problem. Severe abdominal pain and vomiting may sometimes indicate a medical emergency. Always seek medical help for symptoms that are persistent or severe.

Upper abdominal pain

Providing there is no nausea or vomiting, apply pressure in the center of the abdomen, under the ribs.

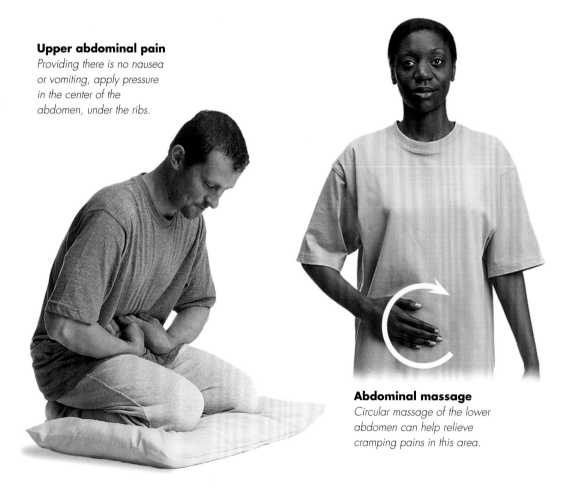

Abdominal massage

Circular massage of the lower abdomen can help relieve cramping pains in this area.

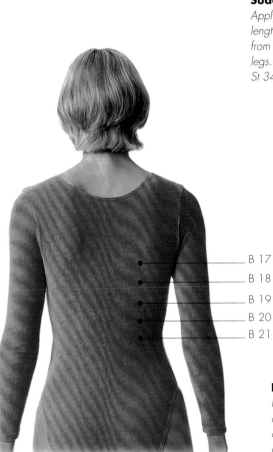

Nausea & vomiting —self-treatment

The classic point used to treat all forms of nausea and vomiting is HP 6. It is easy to apply pressure here yourself.

HP 6

ST 34

ST 36

Sudden abdominal pain

Apply thumb pressure along the length of the Stomach channel from the thigh to the foot on both legs. Pay special attention to St 34, St 36, and St 44.

ST 44

B 17
B 18
B 19
B 20
B 21

Balancing the digestive system

If you have a helper, work on the yu points on the Bladder channel in the middle back can be beneficial. These points relate to the digestive system.

Diarrhea & Constipation

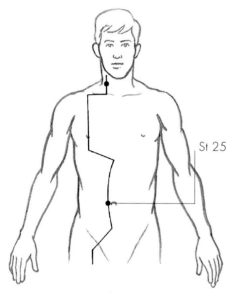

St 25

Large Intestine "Bo" Point
*Also known as St 25, this is situated two
thumb-widths on either side of the navel.
It can help intestinal problems.*

The passage of waste material through the intestines is mainly the concern of the Large Intestine, the yang organ of the Metal element. If this organ is out of balance, the flow of food residues will be speeded up (causing diarrhea) or slowed down (resulting in constipation). Such imbalances often occur as a result of disharmony of related organs having a "domino" effect on the action of the Large Intestine. If you experience any change in bowel habit, report it to your doctor.

Diarrhea

Acute diarrhea is often associated with excessive cold or damp or inadequate yang ki in the Stomach, Spleen, or Kidney channels. Treat the Spleen channel in the foot and leg, giving special emphasis to tsubos Sp 3 (Greater Whiteness) and Sp 4. Do not work the Spleen channel in pregnancy. St 25 has an important regulatory action on the Large Intestine.

Irritable bowel syndrome

This stress-related condition is indicated by alternating bouts of diarrhea and constipation, often accompanied by cramping pains. Breathe deeply and try massaging the lower abdomen using a circular motion for a few minutes.

Constipation

The abdominal area is energized by cv 6, which can stimulate a sluggish, constipated bowel. Shiatsu along the outer arm and hand, emphasizing the Large Intestine and Triple Heater channels, may also be

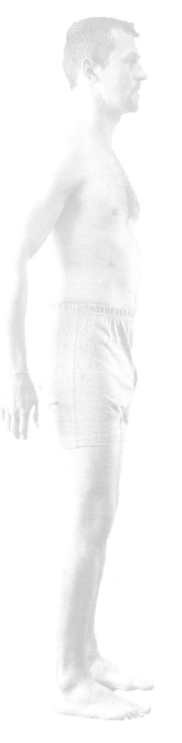

helpful. Pay special attention to LI 4,
(Great Eliminator) which can promote
bowel action. It should never be used in
pregnancy. TH 6 is another effective point
for all three abdominal regions.

Working on the Gallbladder and Liver
channels on the sides of the body and
legs assists movement throughout the
body. Pay particular attention to GB 34
(Yang Mound Spring), which helps to
relax muscle spasm and may relieve
constipation. Li 3 (Great Pouring) helps
the distribution of Liver ki, promoting
regularity in all body functions.

A partner can help by working on the yu
points on the Bladder channel in the lower
back (B 23 to B 32), which influence the
processes of elimination.

TREATMENT ROUTINE
Imbalances of the Large Intestine organ, generally manifested as constipation or diarrhea, often occur as a result of disharmony of related organs. Most of the treatments for specific tsubos shown here can be self-administered. Work on the relevant points once or twice a day. Maintain an adequate fluid intake for both conditions, and for constipation be sure to include a high proportion of fruit, vegetables, and whole grains in your diet.

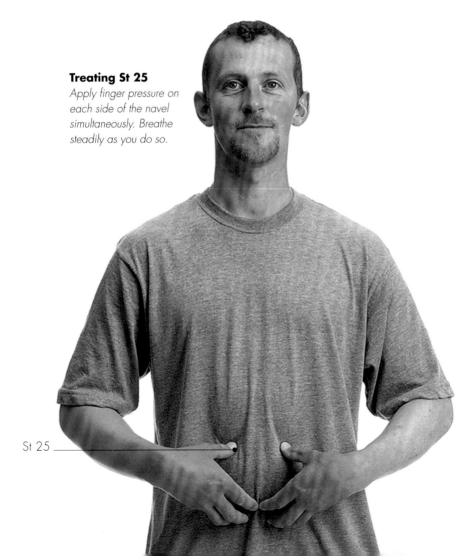

Treating St 25
Apply finger pressure on each side of the navel simultaneously. Breathe steadily as you do so.

St 25

Constipation

Shiatsu treatment of the Gallbladder and Liver channels along the side of the body is beneficial.

Diarrhea

For loose or frequent bowel movements, apply finger or thumb pressure to Sp 3 and Sp 4. Do not use these points in pregnancy.

Sp 3

Sp 4

B 25

B 30

Balancing the bowels

Work on the Bladder channel in the lower back can have a beneficial effect on the action of the bowels. Work from B 25 to B 30.

Joint Problems

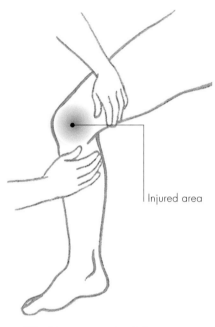

Working around a joint

When a joint has been injured, do not apply pressure directly to the area. Instead, gently thumb around the joint.

Injured area

Joint pain and stiffness may result from a long-standing (chronic) problem, such as osteoarthritis, or they may arise from an acute injury or strain. Shiatsu can ease both types of problem by promoting the free flow of ki through the affected part. This relieves what shiatsu practitioners refer to as "painful blockage," which occurs when damage to a joint blocks the channels that run through it.

Injury

Always seek prompt medical advice following injury to a joint where there is a possibility of dislocation or a broken bone. Do not work directly on a joint that has recently been injured or is currently painful or inflamed. Instead treat the relevant channels in other areas on the same side of the body. Observe the precise location of any pain and use this information to decide where to apply treatment. If the injury is, for example, on the inner aspect of the knee, work on the inner leg above and below the painful area.

Liver & Gallbladder

The Liver and Gallbladder are organs of the Wood element. They are linked to the ligaments and tendons and have a generally restorative effect on the joints. Work on these channels to promote healing of sprains and strains. GB 34 has a particular association with all the paired joints of the body (for example, knees, ankles, and shoulders). Work on GB 40

(Ruined Mound) can also help to relieve ankle, knee, and hip pain. Treatment of GB 30 (Jumping Circle) is often effective for the relief of hip pain.

Kidney & Bladder

If joint problems arise from bone weakness, as can occur with osteoporosis, it may be helpful to strengthen Kidney and Bladder ki. These organs of the Water element are associated with bone health. Work on the lower back, emphasizing the yu points on the Bladder channel and treat the Kidney channel in the inner leg. B 11 in the upper back is a special tsubo for strengthening the bones. You may need a partner to apply pressure to some of these points.

Joint Flexibility

The Makko-ho exercises described on pages 40–55 help to improve and maintain joint flexibility.

TREATMENT ROUTINE

For acute joint problems, your primary concern is to free the flow of ki through the affected joint. Work gently with your thumbs around, but not over, the joint. Follow the course of any channels that pass through it. Later you may wish to work on distant points of the Gallbladder channel that help the long-term healing of the joints, and those on the Bladder channel that strengthen the bones.

Knee injury

In this type of injury it is usually better if someone else carries out shiatsu treatment. Ask your helper to apply palm and thumb pressure around the knee area, working outward up and down the leg.

Palming below the knee

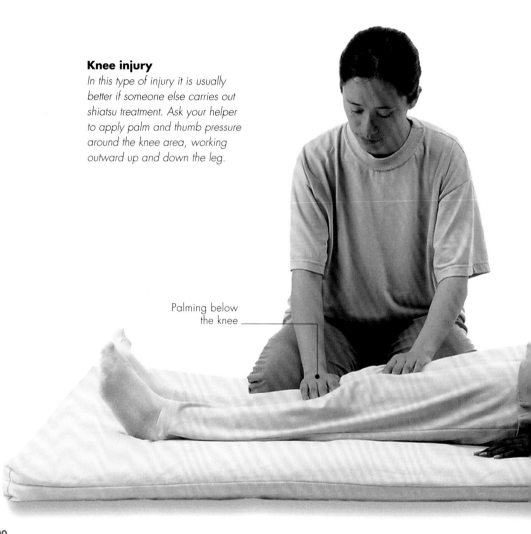

Bone strengthening

Where bone weakness is suspected (e.g. in osteoporosis or accompanying arthritis), ask a helper to treat B 11 in the upper back.

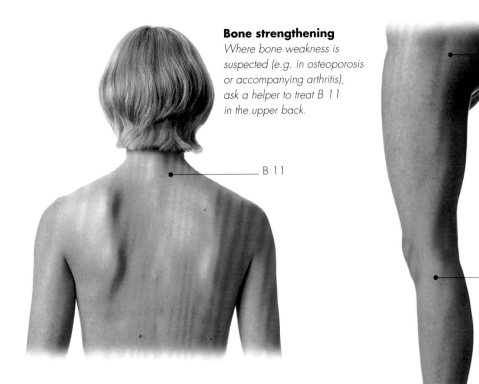

B 11

GB 30

GB 34

GB 40

General joint disorders

The Liver and Gallbladder channels are the most important for joint function. It is helpful to treat these whatever your joint problem. In particular, apply pressure along the Gallbladder channel from the hip to the ankle, giving special emphasis to GB 30, GB 34, and GB 40.

Urinary Problems

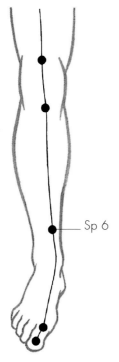

Three Yin Meeting
*Spleen 6 occurs on the inside of the
lower leg at the junction of three yin channels:
Spleen, Kidney, and Liver.*

n TCM, urine is controlled by the
Bladder and Kidneys, the organs of the
Water element. The Bladder transforms
waste fluids from the Lungs, Large
Intestine, and Small Intestine into urine.
The Kidneys regulate water levels in the
body. Urinary problems are not
necessarily the result of imbalances in
these organs. A tendency to urinary tract
infections may arise from general
weakness of ki and blood. Painful,
frequent urination with pain in the lower
abdomen or back can be a sign of a
serious bladder or kidney infection and
needs to be evaluated by a doctor. Such
problems may originate in poor diet,
emotional trauma, or dampness and heat
that deplete Spleen ki, which governs
the transformation of ki into blood. This
type of underlying problem may be
best treated via the Spleen channel.

Painful urination

For painful, frequent urination with pain
in the lower abdomen and back, ask a
partner to treat the yu points on the
Bladder channel in the lower back and
sacral area (B 27–34). This has a
stimulating effect on the organs involved
with urination. Pressure applied to B 60
may help to relieve pain on urination. The
abdominal points CV 3 (Utmost Middle)
and St 29 have a strengthening effect on
the system as a whole.

Sp 6

Provided you are not pregnant, you may also apply pressure to Sp 6, either separately or as part of a full treatment of the Spleen channel. This tsubo, also known as Three Yin Meeting, is an important point at the convergence of the three yin channels that flow through the lower leg: Spleen, Kidneys, and Liver. These channels flow to the pelvic region, so Sp 6 is helpful for urinary problems and has a powerful regulatory effect on all reproductive functions.

Fluids

In addition to the shiatsu treatments described here, be sure to drink plenty of clear fluids while you have symptoms of urinary tract problems. This helps to flush out any infection and dilutes the urine so that any burning pain is lessened. Consult a doctor in all cases.

Lower Back Treatment

Shiatsu treatment of the lower back area can benefit those suffering from urinary tract problems, see pages 108–11.

TREATMENT ROUTINE

To relieve urinary tract problems, work the points suggested for self-administration several times a day until symptoms abate. Treatment of the Bladder channel yu points in the lower back and sacrum, for which you need a helper, can be effective when done less frequently. If you do not have anyone to give you shiatsu, practice the makko-ho stretches for the Bladder and Kidneys on pages 50–51.

Strengthening the system
To boost the urinary system as a whole, apply finger pressure to CV 3 in the center of the lower abdomen four thumb-widths below the navel. Pressure on St 29 may also be helpful in this way.

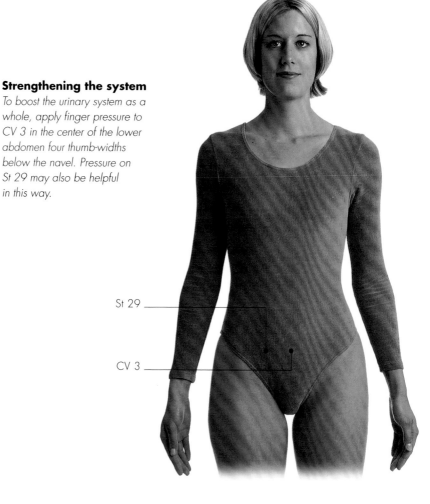

St 29

CV 3

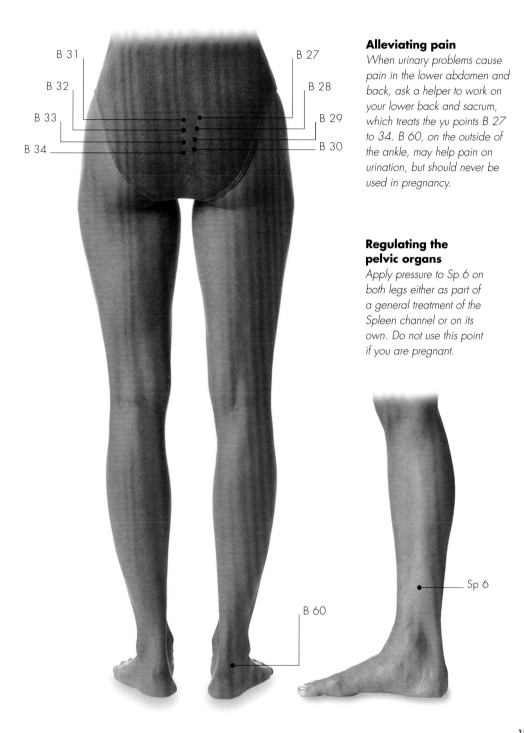

B 31
B 32
B 33
B 34

B 27
B 28
B 29
B 30

B 60

Sp 6

Alleviating pain

When urinary problems cause pain in the lower abdomen and back, ask a helper to work on your lower back and sacrum, which treats the yu points B 27 to 34. B 60, on the outside of the ankle, may help pain on urination, but should never be used in pregnancy.

Regulating the pelvic organs

Apply pressure to Sp 6 on both legs either as part of a general treatment of the Spleen channel or on its own. Do not use this point if you are pregnant.

Reproductive System

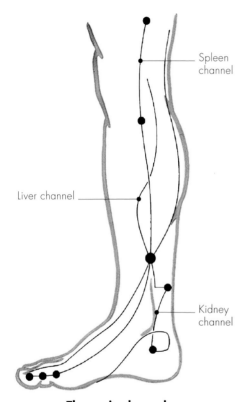

Three yin channels

The three channels of the inner leg are the most important for the regulation of the reproductive system.

Spleen channel

Liver channel

Kidney channel

The Spleen, Liver, and Kidneys govern the health of reproductive organs and processes in both men and women. This section is concerned with symptoms affecting the female reproductive organs and menstrual cycle. The key point for all symptoms relating to menstruation is Sp 6, which should be treated in all cases, provided you are certain you are not pregnant.

Premenstrual problems

Irritability, breast tenderness, and bloating are the result of inactive, or stagnant, Liver ki, causing imbalances in the Stomach and Spleen. Treat the Heart Protector channel to combat psychological symptoms, and HP 6 and HP 7 for bloating and breast tenderness. Work on all the leg channels is also beneficial.

Menstrual pain

Pain that is worse at the start of menstruation may be alleviated by working on Li 3 (Great Pouring) and Li 2 (Walk Between). Palm pressure on CV 6 and 4 may also be soothing. Work the whole sacral area and the Bladder tsubos B 23 and B 32 to treat back pain that occurs toward the end of menstruation.

Blood loss

Use firm finger pressure on CV 4 to treat heavy blood loss or abnormally long periods. Strengthen the Spleen by working along the whole channel in the inner leg, paying particular attention to Sp 10 (Sea of Blood), which inhibits bleeding, Sp 6, and Sp 1. Treating Li 1 may be helpful.

Menopause

Many women suffer a variety of unpleasant symptoms such as excessive sweating, mood changes, and disturbed sleep around the time that menstruation ceases permanently. In TCM such problems are seen as the result of disharmony of Heart and Kidneys. Heart imbalances may be regulated by working on H 7 (Mind Door) and H 6. Regular treatment of the Kidney channel in the leg and ankle is also helpful. Pay special attention to K 1 (Bubbling Spring), K 6 (Shining Sea), and K 7. Treatment of Sp 10 may also be helpful for cooling the hot flashes that occur during menopause.

TREATMENT ROUTINE

All problems relating to the menstrual cycle benefit from treatment of Sp 6. Work on the tsubos and channels concerned with your specific problem as appropriate. The frequency with which you carry out treatment depends on the severity of symptoms. Once daily may be enough if your symptoms are mild. However, if menstrual pain is severe, treat the suggested tsubos every few hours. Consult your doctor if severe pain is unrelieved by treatment.

Relieving pain

Ask a helper to apply pressure to the yu points of the lower back (B 23 and B 32). You can self-administer CV 4 and CV 6 (see opposite). Work on the Liver channel tsubos on the foot, Li 3 and Li 2 (see page 203), can also help relieve pain.

Sp 10

Stemming menstrual flow

Apply firm pressure to CV 4 (see opposite), then treat the Spleen channel on the inner leg, giving emphasis to Sp 10, Sp 6 and Sp 1.

B 23

B 32

Sp 6

K 7

K 6

Sp 1

K 1

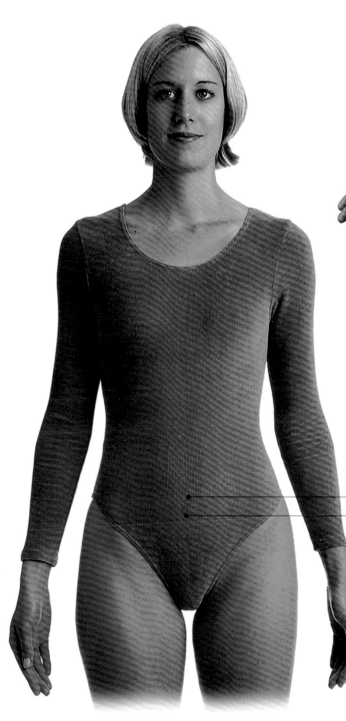

H 6

H 7

Menopausal symptoms

Alleviate excessive sweating and hot flashes by working the Heart channel in the arm, especially H 6 and H 7. Treatment of the Kidney channel, especially K 1 (see also page 200), K 6, and K 7 may also help. Regular work on Sp 10 (see left) can be of benefit in reducing hot flashes.

CV 6

CV 4

Anxiety & Insomnia

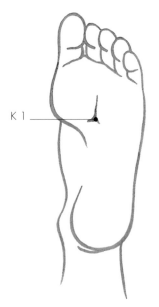

Bubbling Spring

The first point on the Kidney channel is both calming and strengthening in cases of anxiety.

K 1

Anxiety and the associated difficulty sleeping are often the result of excess yang energy, particularly in the upper part of the body. These symptoms may also be caused by a lack of blood or nourishment in the lower part of the body. Excess yang energy may also lead to feelings of lightheadedness. These treatments will help disperse it.

Dispersing yang

Shiatsu treatment of the head and face helps to disperse excess yang. This should be followed by treatment of the feet and ankles to draw the energy downward. The tsubos K 6 (Shining Sea) and K 1 (Bubbling Spring) are particularly calming. Earth energy is lacking in people suffering from anxiety, and these people often suffer from digestive disturbances related to Stomach and Spleen. Work on these channels in the legs to reconnect with the Earth and help you see your problems in proportion. HP 6, CV 12, and CV 14 may soothe anxiety-related digestive problems.

Heart

Imbalance of the Heart is also a common cause of restlessness and agitation. Treatment of the tsubo H 7 (Mind Door) has a wonderfully soothing effect and has the advantage of being conveniently located for self-treatment.

Liver

When stress related to work or other life events leads to feelings of anxiety, this may indicate a lack of energy in the

Wood element and its related organ, the Liver. The Liver governs planning and creativity, attributes that help you deal with life's challenges. Boosting this energy by working on Li 3 may help you cope with life's everyday demands.

Gallbladder & Large Intestine

Repeated stress can build tension in the neck and shoulders, causing headaches. Relieve these symptoms by working on the shoulder channels, emphasizing GB 20 and GB 21, and by putting pressure on the *yintang* point between the brows. Supplement this by paying attention to LI 4, which helps disperse blocked energy in the neck and shoulders.

Stimulants

Anxiety and insomnia are exacerbated by excessive amounts of stimulants (see pages 60–61). For the shiatsu treatment to be effective, you must minimize your intake.

TREATMENT ROUTINE

A tendency to become anxious, regarded in shiatsu as a manifestation of excess yang energy, is often a longstanding problem. Try to build appropriate shiatsu treatments into your daily routine. You may want to work on Li 3 in the morning to help you prepare for the day's challenges, and on calming points such as κ 1 in the evening to help you relax for sleep. Devise your own self-treatment program to suit your needs.

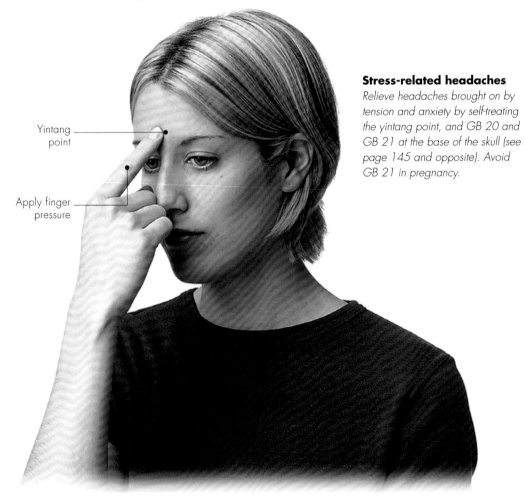

Yintang point

Apply finger pressure

Stress-related headaches
Relieve headaches brought on by tension and anxiety by self-treating the yintang point, and GB 20 and GB 21 at the base of the skull (see page 145 and opposite). Avoid GB 21 in pregnancy.

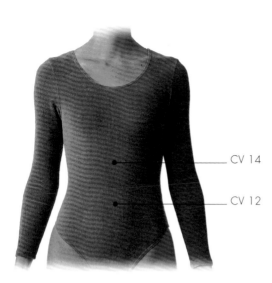

CV 14

CV 12

Li 3

Anxiety-related digestive problems

Apply finger pressure to CV 12 and to CV 14, which is located 8 finger-widths above the navel.

Boosting your ability to cope

Stimulate your power to deal with problems and plan your life by working on the Liver channel, and Li 3 in particular. This is located on the top of the foot at the point where the bones of the first and second toes merge.

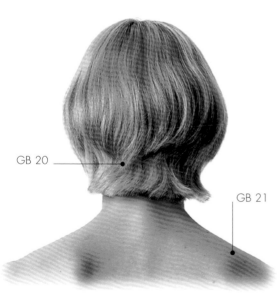

GB 20

GB 21

Anxiety-related neck & shoulder tension

Disperse tension in the neck caused by stress by treating the Gallbladder points in this area: GB 20 and 21. Do not treat GB 21 during pregnancy.

Tiredness & Weakness

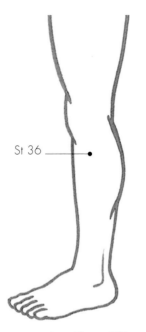

St 36

Leg Three Miles

St 36 is an energizing point for the whole system. It helps the Stomach and Spleen extract ki from food.

Tiredness, lethargy, weakness, and low spirits (depression) are in shiatsu terms all related to low ki— lack of vital energy. This can have many underlying causes that can be addressed by shiatsu treatment. However, do not forget to look at all aspects of your lifestyle—make sure that you are eating a nourishing diet and are achieving a healthy balance between exercise and rest. Seek help and medical advice from your doctor if you are experiencing severe or prolonged depression.

Lungs

Since much of our ki is derived from air, a priority is to stimulate the Lungs and promote deeper breathing. The Lungs are also associated with grief. If the Lung energy is out of balance, depression and negativity are likely to occur. Practice the makko-ho exercises for the Lungs described on pages 42–43 every morning. If you have someone to help you, shiatsu pressure on the upper chest and shoulders in the supine position can be effective in stimulating the Heart and Lungs. Pay special attention to Lu 1 (Central Residence), which promotes the downward flow of Lung energy. It is possible to stimulate this point yourself if you have nobody to help you. Follow the arms and shoulders routine described on pages 126–27 and apply pressure to cv 17, which improves breathing and strengthens ki in the chest area. Press this point yourself, or ask a partner.

Exhaustion

For physical or emotional exhaustion, finger or palm pressure on CV 6. This will give a boost to ki and yang energy, encourages deep, abdominal breathing.

Depression

If depression is the primary problem, include a thorough working of the Lung, Heart Protector, and Heart channels in the arm. Give special emphasis to Lu 7. Some types of depression in which frustration is predominant—perhaps from failure to achieve goals and consequent low self-esteem—benefit from work on the Liver channel in the legs.

Feeling cold

A tendency to feel cold, particularly in the hands and feet, is common when overall ki is depleted. Treatment of St 36 has an invigorating effect.

Caution

If you experience prolonged or severe depression, seek advice from your doctor.

TREATMENT ROUTINE

The Lungs, which govern the intake of air ki, are the most important organ for ensuring overall physical and mental vitality. Get the most out of shiatsu for tiredness, lethargy, and related symptoms by timing your treatment to coincide with the time of day when Lung energy is strongest: during the early morning. Enjoy the energizing effect of the morning light and compensate by going to bed early.

Alleviating depression
Work the Lung channel as a whole, but pay special attention to Lu 7.

Increasing energy
Give your energy levels a boost by applying pressure to CV 17 and Lu 1. Treatment of these points improvies breathing and strengthens Lung ki.

Combating tiredness
Apply finger or palm pressure to CV 6 to increase yang energy throughout the body.

Lu 7

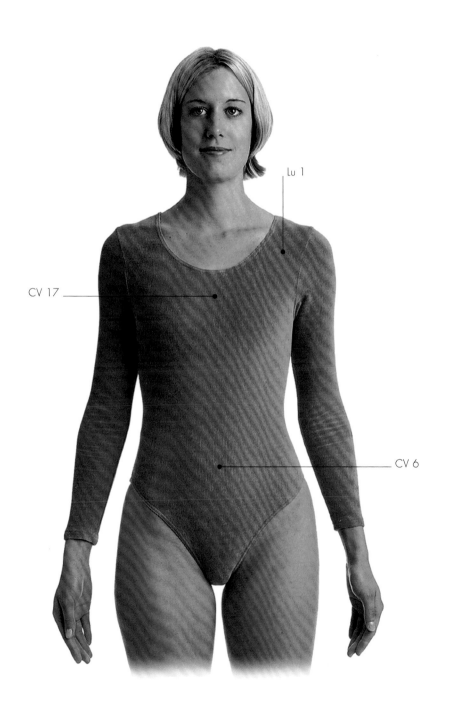

Lu 1

CV 17

CV 6

Back Problems

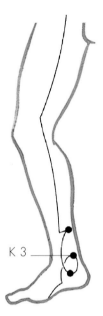

K 3

Low Kidney energy

Back pain is often related to depleted Kidney ki. Work on K 3 provides a rapid boost.

Back pain is one of the most common health problems. The physiological causes include poor posture, strain, and degenerative conditions, such as osteoarthritis. Orthodox treatments often provide only partial relief and complementary therapies, including shiatsu, may bring about lasting improvements. Get a medical assessment of your back pain before applying shiatsu. Seek immediate medical advice if pain is accompanied by numbness or weakness in any limb, or if there is a loss of bladder control.

Chronic pain

In shiatsu terms, chronic back pain, especially in the lumbar area, may be caused by a lack of ki in the Kidney channel, depleted by excessive physical exertion over a long period, or an inherently weak constitution. Some problems in the back relate to the joints between the vertebrae.

Shiatsu along the Bladder channel helps to relieve muscle spasm in the back—a prime cause of pain. Treat the Governing Vessel to address low energy in the Kidney channel. Ask a partner to apply positive but gentle pressure by working with relaxed fingertips along the spine, feeling for the tsubos in the spaces between the vertebrae. In addition, practice the makko-ho exercise for the Kidney and Bladder channels. The late afternoon and early evening, when Kidney energy is at its peak, are the best times for this.

Acute onset

When back pain is of sudden onset, avoid treating the back area directly. Work on the Bladder tsubos on the feet and ankles to strengthen the back. B 60 and B 62 are most effective. K 3 boosts Kidney ki and alleviates back pain. Further up the leg, B 40 strengthens the back and supports yang energy in the Kidney. SI 3 has a relaxing influence on the muscles of the neck and back and helps to calm the mind after a shock. Located in the hand, this is easily accessible for self-treatment.

Sciatica

Sciatica is pain that originates in the lower back and shoots down the back of the leg. This requires medical investigation, but shiatsu treatment of the Gallbladder channel from GB 30 down the outside of the leg to GB 40 may be helpful in alleviating pain.

TREATMENT ROUTINE

When back pain is acute (of recent onset), rest is key to allow the muscles time to relax, and to permit depleted ki to be replenished — an important aspect of recovery. While you rest, have a helper work on tsubos away from your back. When pain has abated, have shiatsu treatment of the back itself. In the long term, examine your lifestyle to prevent a recurrence of the problem.

Low back pain
Apply pressure to GV 26. This reviving point is actually located on the inside of your upper lip. Finger pressure can be exerted externally over the point. The best way to do this is to lean over onto your finger, allowing the weight of your head to provide the force.

External finger pressure to GV 26

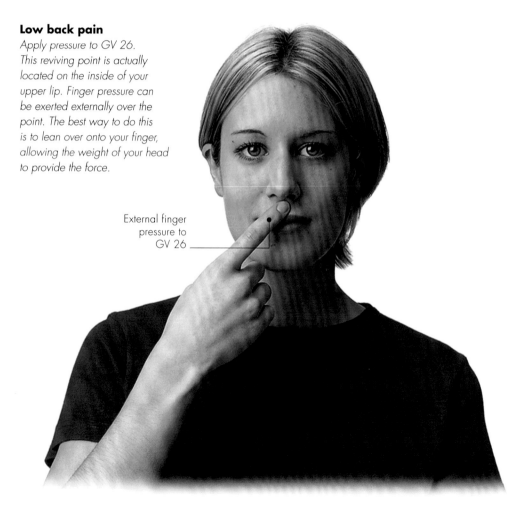

Back strengthening

Regular work on the tsubos of the Bladder channel located on the foot—B 62 and B 60—is often effective for strengthening the back after strain or injury. B 40, at the back of the knee, is a well-known tsubo for helping the back to withstand strain.

B 40

B 60

B 62

Muscle relaxant

Back pain is often associated with stiff muscles in the back. Firm pressure applied to SI 3 can help to relax the back and neck.

Gallbladder channel

Supporting sciatica treatment

Treat the Gallbladder channel from the hip to the ankle to help relieve the symptoms of sciatica. Carefully work into any tsubos you encounter.

SI 3

Eyes & Ears

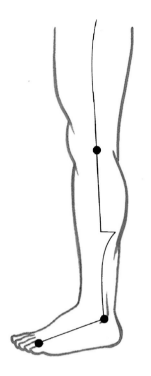

Gallbladder channel

This is the yang channel of the Wood element, and it exerts influence over the eyes and eyesight.

The senses of sight and hearing are among the chief means by which we take in information about the outside world. The eyes and ears are constantly at work, assimilating and sorting a constant stream of stimuli during our waking hours. When they do not function properly or are a source of pain or discomfort, it is particularly distressing and disorienting, because our communication with the world around us is disrupted. In all cases of pain or impaired vision or hearing, seek medical advice. Use shiatsu treatments to support any treatments prescribed by your doctor.

Eye and ear problems are often improved by local treatment of the tsubos of the head and face. This helps to clear any blockages in the nearby channels and allows the free flow of energy to restore normal function. Use finger pressure to work around affected areas.

Eyes

The eyes and vision are associated with the Wood element and by extension with the Liver and Gallbladder. Locally effective tsubos include B 1 (Eye Brightness), B 2 (Gathering Bamboo), TH 23 (Silk Bamboo Hollow), GB 1 (Orbit Bone), and St 2. For general strengthening of the eyes and eyesight, work on the Gallbladder channel in the lower leg. Tired eyes that have difficulty focusing benefit from treatment of Li 3 in the foot. GB 20 (Wind Pool) can also help clear vision. Pressure on LI 4 is often effective for eye inflammation caused by hay fever and other allergic conditions. The Kidneys govern the processes of aging. Regular work on K 3 may benefit older people who suffer from degenerative eye conditions.

Ears

The ears and hearing are linked to the Water element and its related organs: the Kidneys and Bladder. Hearing loss and ringing in the ears may result from Kidney disharmony and may therefore benefit from regular treatment of the Kidney channels. An earache is more likely to be the result of external influences such as exposure to wind. Treatment of the tsubos in the ear area can be of help in such cases. These tsubos include TH 17 (Wind Screen), SI 19 (Listening Palace), and TH 3 (Middle Islet).

TREATMENT ROUTINE
Before and after using shiatsu to treat the eye area, it is helpful to "palm" both eyes together. This is soothing and relaxing for the eye muscles and makes the eyes more receptive to the effects of shiatsu pressure. Repeat local treatment of the eye or ear area every hour or so while symptoms persist. Work on the distant points for strengthening the system once or twice a day.

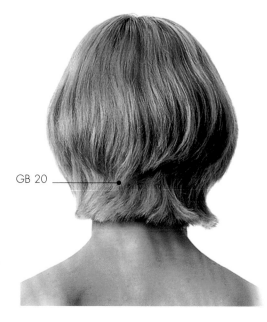

GB 20

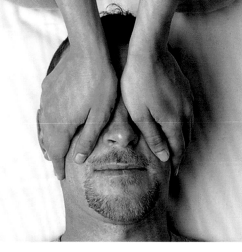

Problems in eye area

Treating GB 20 at the base of the skull between the bands of muscle at the back and sides of the neck may help to clear vision.

Palming

Palming is a soothing way to relax your eyes. You can do it yourself or have a helper do it for you. Place the center of each palm over one eye. Keep your palms over the eyes for a few moments.

Local eye treatment

Pay special attention to the points shown here, using gentle, positive pressure.

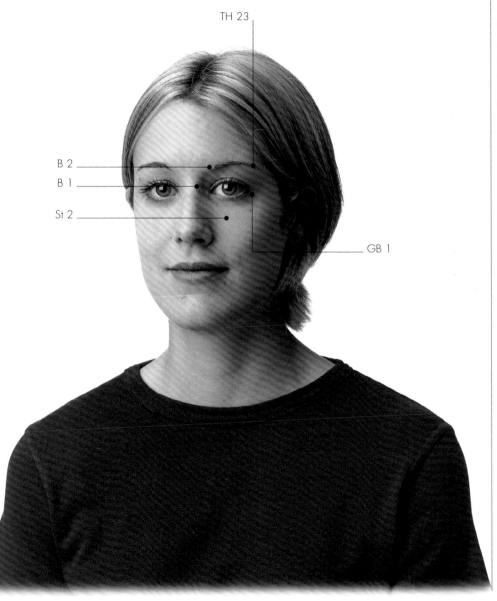

TH 23

B 2

B 1

St 2

GB 1

GLOSSARY

The glossary contains technical terms that the reader may encounter when reading this book or in other contexts. If you do not find the information you need here, try the general index (pages 222–223).

Acupressure
The manipulation of energy flow in the body through pressure on specific points on the energy channels (meridians).

Ahshi points
Points on the body that are particularly sensitive to either touch or pressure as a result of muscular tension or disrupted energy flow.

Anma
The traditional form of Japanese massage, from which shiatsu is in part derived.

Cold
An external climatic condition that in Traditional Chinese Medicine, can adversely affect the internal organs, especially the Bladder and Kidneys. Cold may cause fevers, shivering, muscle cramps, and/or joint pain.

Cun
The traditional unit of measurement used for locating specific points on the channels. One cun is roughly the width of the thumb of the person in question.

Dampness
An external climatic condition (see Cold) that primarily affects the Stomach and Spleen, leading to heaviness, numbness, and swelling particularly of the lower body. It can also produce excessive, watery mucus.

Do-In
A system of exercises for improving the flow of ki.

Dryness
An external climatic condition (see Cold) that primarily affects the Large Intestine and Lungs, leading to dryness of the mouth, throat, and skin, and constipation. It may also cause a dry cough.

Fire
An external climatic condition (see Cold) that is also known as heat. It primarily affects the Heart, Heart Protector, Small Intestine, and Triple Heater. Fire can cause high fever, a red face, sweating, thirst, restlessness, and irritability.

Futon
A traditional Japanese mattress made from layers of cotton wadding. A futon provides a firm but comfortable surface, which is ideal for giving shiatsu.

Hara
The Japanese term for the belly. In shiatsu the hara is important as the physical center of gravity and also the energy center of the body.

Heat
See Fire.

Ki
The Japanese form of the Chinese qi or chi, the vital energy of the universe that flows throughout the body. Shiatsu aims to enhance well-being by harmonizing this energy flow.

Lumbar
Commonly known as the "small of the back", this term refers to the area most commonly affected by back pain. Anatomically the lumbar spine comprises the last five vertebrae before the sacrum.

Meridian
A term often used for the channels in the body through which energy, or ki, flows.

Sacrum
The large, flat area of bone at the base of the spine.

Tanden
Also known as the "sea of ki," the center of the hara (see above) located three finger-widths below the navel.

Thorax
The chest and upper back. The 12 thoracic vertebrae are connected to the ribs.

Tsubo
The Japanese term for a point at which energy gathers and at which its flow through the body can be influenced by pressure. Many tsubos are located at the classic points on the energy channels used in acupuncture. But additional tsubos can also be found elsewhere.

Wind
An external climatic condition (see Cold) that primarily affects the Gallbladder and Liver, but may also have more widespread consequences. Wind can cause sudden and violent symptoms, such as headaches, dizziness, a streaming nose and sneezing, muscle spasms, and aversion to wind.

Yin-Yang
The concept of all things being composed of a balance of opposing, but complementary qualities. This idea is fundamental to Chinese medicine, which in all its forms seeks to harmonize the interaction of Yin and Yang energy in the body.

Zen
A form of Buddhism that is prevalent in Japan. Zen shiatsu, developed by Shizuto Masunaga, is a form of shiatsu that incorporates ideas drawn from Traditional Chinese Medicine and the spiritual approaches learned from Zen Buddhism.

USEFUL ADDRESSES

US

American Organization for Bodywork Therapies of Asia
AOBTA National Office,
P.O. BOX 343, West Berlin
NJ 08091
Tel: (836) 809 2953
office@aobta.org

American College of Acupuncture and Oriental Medicine
9100 Park West Drive
Houston, TX 77063
Tel: (713) 780 9777
www.acaom.edu

American Association of Acupuncture and Oriental Medicine
P.O. BOX 96503 #44114
Washington D.C.
20090-6503
admin@aaaomonline.org
www.aaaomonline.org

American Holistic Health Association
P.O. Box 17400
Ananheim, CA 92817
Tel: 714 779 6152
mail@ahha.org
www.ahha.org

UK

Shiatsu Society (UK)
P.O. BOX 4580
Rugby, CV21 9EL
UK
Tel: 01788 547 900
Fax: 01788 547 111
admin@shiatsusociety.org
www.shiatsusociety.org

The Shiatsu College
Tel: 0800 690 6349
shiatsucollege.co.uk

EUROPE

The European Shiatsu Federation
Alternativ Akademin
Rundelsgränd 2 B, 753 12,
Uppsala, Sweden
info@
europeanshiatsufederation.eu
www.
europeanshiatsufederation.eu

AUSTRALIA

Australian Traditional Medicine Society
Suite 12/27 Bank Street
Meadowbank, New South
Wales, 2114
Tel: 1 800 456855
info@atms.com.au

IRELAND

Shiatsu Society of Ireland
admin@shiatsusociety.org
shiatsusocietyireland.org

FURTHER READING

Beresford-Cooke, Carola, *Shiatsu Theory and Practice*, Singing Dragon, 2016.

Jarmey, Chris, *Shiatsu Foundation Course*, Godsfield Press, 1999.

Jarmey, Chris and Tindall, John, *Acupressure for Common Ailments*, Gaia Books, 1991.

Kaptchuk, Ted, *Chinese Medicine: The Web that has no Weaver*, Rider, 1993.

Liechti, Elaine, *The Complete Illustrated Guide to Shiatsu*, Element Books, 1998.

Lundberg, Paul, *The New Book of Shiatsu*, Gaia Books, 2014.

Masunaga, Shizuto, *Zen Shiatsu*, Japan Publications, 1977.

Namikoshi, Tokujiro, *The Complete Book of Shiatsu Therapy*, Japan Publications, 1987.

Pooley, Nicola, *Shiatsu, A Step-by-Step Guide*, Element Books, 1998.

Serizawa, Katsusuke, *Tsubo: Vital Points for Oriental Therapy*, Japan Publications, 1976.

Tsu, Lao (trans. Man Ho Kwok, Martin Palmer, and Jay Ramsey), *Tao Te Ching*, Element Books, 1993.

Veith, Ilza (trans.), *The Yellow Emperor's Classic of Internal Medicine*, University of California Press, 1966.

Williams, Tom, *Chinese Medicine*, Element Books, 1995.

INDEX

ACKNOWLEDGMENTS

The publisher would like to thank Deborah Fielding
for reading and commenting on the text, and Martha's Barn in
Brighton, UK for the loan of the shiatsu mats.
Cathy Meeus would like to thank Paul Lundberg for sharing his knowledge.

PICTURE ACKNOWLEDGMENTS

The publisher would like to thank the following for permission to reproduce
copyright material:

Alamy/ Image Source: 175; Lumi Images: 67

Getty/ George Doyle: 99

Images Colour Library/ AGE Fotostock: 18T

iStock/ dja65: 22TR; omgimages: 11; Squaredpixels: 35; vellena: 2

Shutterstock/ bento42894: 14T; canadastock: 18B; D7INAMI7S: 19MR;
KreativKolors: 13; kubais: 22M; Lepas: 19TL; Sarah Marchant: 22BR;
Alexander Mazurkevich: 19TR; Sementer: 22BL; Tim UR: 19ML;
warat42: 19BR; Edward Westmacott: 19BL; xpixel: 22TL